NOT in BIP pb. 09

O9-CFU-527

CIRCLE
OF MADNESS

Robert Perrucci is a Professor of Sociology at Purdue University. He is the co-author of *Profession Without Community* (1968), and co-editor of *The Triple Revolution* (1968), *The Engineers and the Social System* (1969), and *The Triple Revolution Emerging* (1971). He has published articles in the areas of social stratification, complex organizations, and social problems, and is currently completing research on the social processes involved in commitment to a mental hospital.

Robert Perrucci

CIRCLE
OF MADNESS

On Being Insane
and Institutionalized
in America

A SPECTRUM BOOK

PRENTICE-HALL, INC., *Englewood Cliffs, New Jersey*

Library of Congress Cataloging in Publication Data

PERRUCCI, ROBERT.
  Circle of madness.

  (A Spectrum book)
  Includes bibliographical references.
  1. Psychiatric hospitals—Sociological aspects.
2. Psychiatric hospital care—United States.
3. Psychology, Pathological. I. Title.
RC439.P43   362.2'04'25   74–23535
ISBN 0–13–133884–6
ISBN 0–13–133876–5 pbk.

PRENTICE-HALL INTERNATIONAL, INC. (LONDON)
PRENTICE-HALL OF AUSTRALIA PTY., LTD. (SYDNEY)
PRENTICE-HALL OF CANADA, LTD. (TORONTO)
PRENTICE-HALL OF INDIA PRIVATE LIMITED (NEW DELHI)
PRENTICE-HALL OF JAPAN, INC. (TOKYO)

To
Louis Schneider
who first told me about a dreamer's journey

Contents

Acknowledgments

Acknowledgment is gratefully made to the following:

To the *American Sociological Review*, for permission to reprint "Social Distance Strategies and Intraorganizational Stratification," 28, 6 (December 1963), 951–62.

To The William Alanson White Psychiatric Foundation, for permission to reprint "Social Distance, Bargaining Power, and Compliance with Roles on a Hospital Ward," *Psychiatry* 29, 1 (February 1966), 42–55. © 1966 The William Alanson White Psychiatric Foundation.

To Houghton Mifflin Company, for permission to reprint "Heroes and Hopelessness in a Total Institution," and "Social Processes in Psychiatric Decisions," from *Explorations in Sociology and Counseling*, Donald A. Hansen, ed. (Boston, 1969).

To Little, Brown & Co., Inc., for permission to quote from *The Discovery of the Asylum*, by David J. Rothman (Boston, 1971) © 1971 Little, Brown & Co., Inc.

To Pantheon Books/A Division of Random House, Inc., for permission to quote from *Madness and Civilization*, by Michel Foucault, translated by Richard Howard (New York, 1965) © 1965 Random House, Inc.

To Harper and Row Publishers, Inc., for permission to quote from *Madness in Society*, by George Rosen (New York, 1967) © 1967 Harper and Row Publishers, Inc.

To University of Chicago Press, for permission to quote from *Pop-*

ular Religion, by Louis Schneider and Sanford M. Dornbusch (Chicago, 1958) © 1958 University of Chicago.

To The Free Press, for permission to quote from *Suicide,* by Emile Durkheim (New York, 1951) © 1951 The Free Press.

To The Free Press, for permission to quote from *Essays in Sociological Theory,* by Talcott Parsons (New York, 1954) © 1954 The Free Press.

Preface

This book is about life in a mental hospital as I saw it during a year of fieldwork. Its central purpose is to examine the way in which becoming mentally ill, being mentally ill, and becoming normal again are related to communal definitions and relationships. I maintain the point of view that mental patients are victims rather than disease carriers, and that patients and their caretakers are bound together by a shared stigma.

It is my firm belief that most patients in mental hospitals could get along quite well outside hospitals if they could live in supportive family settings with sufficient resources to sustain someone who experiences problems with living. Only in a society that worships efficiency is it easier to expel persons who have difficulty "fitting" than to adjust to the needs of these members.

Substantial sections of Chapters Four, Five, Six, and Seven have appeared elsewhere. These materials have been rewritten or expanded to fit the chapters written especially for this book.

I am especially grateful to Carolyn Perrucci, who allowed me to interfere repeatedly with her own busy schedule to ask for her advice on and critical reading of the manuscript.

Portions of this manuscript were read in article form by Louis Schneider, Arthur Stinchcombe, James Beshers, Ephraim Mizruchi, and Donald Hansen. I gratefully acknowledge their constructive comments. Appreciation is also expressed to Jeanne Plumb for her conscientious work in preparation of the manuscript.

Finally, I would like to thank Michael Hunter of Prentice-Hall for his encouragement and cooperation on this project.

ROBERT PERRUCCI
West Lafayette, Indiana

CIRCLE
OF MADNESS

I

BECOMING DIFFERENT

1

The Communal Nature
of Madness

An examination of the history of mental illness would lead us to consider the place of the mentally ill, the beliefs about the causes for their condition, and the "treatment" applied to that condition, in relation to the social setting in which they are found. Often such historical writings reveal a variety of exotic, bizarre, and sometimes unbelievable accounts of what people in a particular historical period thought about mental illness and how they dealt with those who were so afflicted. A casual reading of these histories reveals a genuine progress from the prescientific period of ignorant and inhumane treatment of madness, through the Enlightenment, to the modern, scientific era of informed and humane treatment. In short, the histories seem to emphasize and dwell upon the different ways in which the mentally ill have been treated in different eras.

Our purpose here is not to ignore or dispute the existence of important changes in beliefs about mental illness and its treatment, but rather to look beyond the assertions of change and progress to what appear to be relatively constant and stable features of madness in a social context. The mentally ill have been ignored, dehumanized, rediscovered, and then rehumanized so many times in history as to make any simple theory of progress suspect. In addition, the very obvious difference between the ancient practice of expelling madmen from the community (when there was no family to care for them) and the modern practice of committing them to a mental hospital (when there is no family willing to care for them) should not blind us to the similarity of the ultimate objectives—to cast the mad out of the community and separate them from their society.

Popular beliefs and practices about mental illness, as well as the beliefs and practices of those considered experts in such matters, are best understood as the result of composite social, political, and economic events that shape a particular historical period rather than as the extension or elaboration of knowledge and beliefs about mental illness. The growth of the asylum in America as the place where the mentally ill are treated is not simply the triumph of a medical theory about diseases of the mind and how they should be treated. Ideas about the causes and treatment of mental illness have the force of change when they are associated with interest groups seeking such change; and, more often than not, change-oriented movements contain such a strange mixture of motives, goals, and interests that it is difficult to see the end product—the growth of the asylum—as a consequence of a receptivity to new and better knowledge about mental illness.

In this first chapter we shall examine some of the historical variability and stability in the place of the mentally ill in their society. Special attention will be given to the emergence and growth of the asylum (i.e., mental hospital) in America, because this is the particular social invention with which we are concerned. One of the general purposes of this review is to acquaint the reader with the ways in which the mentally ill have been viewed in history. The main purpose, however, is to provide a background against which we shall contrast two fundamentally different and conflicting approaches to mental illness which are dominating the contemporary scene. On the one hand there is the medical community's emphasis upon the individual nature of madness, which sees the mentally ill as carriers of a disease that leads them to become *patients*. On the other hand there is a social science emphasis upon the communal nature of madness, which views the mentally ill as *victims* of external forces that lead them to the madhouse.

PREMODERN CONCEPTIONS: SINNERS AND THE POSSESSED

Available materials on the history of mental illness start with the ancient world of Palestine, Greece, and Rome.[1] Among the Israelites, madness in the general population seems not to have

[1] George Rosen, *Madness in Society* (Chicago: University of Chicago Press, 1968).

received the same kind of consideration given to that exhibited by rulers and prophets. Biblical literature abounds with descriptions of séances, trances, hallucinations, visions, convulsive agitations, voice changes, frenzied leaps, self-lacerations, and assorted "unusual" acts of princes and prophets.[2] Such acts were not judged to be psychopathological, but within the normal boundaries of community expectations of the behavior of those in high places. As Rosen puts it, "When a society regards highly individuals who are able to produce unusual psychological states, such persons will appear."[3]

Those ordinary mortals of ancient Palestine afflicted with madness were either consigned to the care of their families, or if not a threat to the community, allowed to roam the streets freely. Little thought seems to have been given to the medical aspects of madness. According to Rosen, Talmudic teachers attempted to link mental illness with legal and moral transgressions, but the absence of references to the treatment of mental illness in the Talmud would suggest little development of thought about natural "causes" of mental illness. There is, in contrast, some evidence of the use of folk and magical practices designed to cast out the demons of madness.

In ancient Greece and Rome, on the other hand, there were both natural and supernatural explanations of madness. According to prevailing medical views of that time:

Mental abnormality was considered a disease, or a symptom of one, caused in the same way as disease of the body. This view was based on the theory which was used to explain not only mental disease, but disease in general, namely, the humoral theory. According to this doctrine, the body was composed of four humours, blood, phlegm, yellow bile, and black bile, which were produced by physiologic processes in various organs of the body. Furthermore, each humour was endowed with a basic quality, such as heat, cold, dryness, and moistness. Disease developed when internal or external factors produced an excess of one of these humours. The resulting imbalance of these basic qualities acted on organs to produce deleterious effects. Madness, the disease of the mind, was produced in this fashion by excess of a humour. Black bile was a peculiarly potent cause, when present in abundance under certain conditions, of various forces of mental illness, particularly the condition called melancholia.[4]

---

[2] Ibid., Chapter 2.
[3] Ibid., p. 63.
[4] Ibid., p. 74.

Although prevailing medical opinion was that an imbalance of "humours" would lead to madness, general public belief was that madness came from possession by unseen forces such as demons or spirits, or by transgressions against the gods who had the power to inflict madness on a sinner. The belief that madness was linked with the supernatural seems to be responsible for community reactions to the mentally ill. Because spirits and gods were treated with mixed feelings of awe, fear, and mystery, some of these feelings were apparently transferred to those who were possessed by spirits or who were being punished by gods. Although mad, the possessed or the sinners, because of their contact with the gods and spirits, might have extraordinary powers which could influence those with whom they had contact. This set of beliefs and attitudes resulted in a tendency to avoid the mentally ill, to exclude them from social life.

Greek and Roman behavior toward the mentally ill was generally similar to that found among the Israelites. Public responsibility for those afflicted with madness involved mainly such concerns as legal complications and protection of persons and property against those who were considered violent. Although families were expected to care for those who were ill, less fortunate madmen without families were allowed to roam the streets freely. The uncared-for mentally ill, however, were apparently subjected to greater public scorn and abuse in ancient Greece and Rome than in Palestine.

What we find, then, from this brief examination of the mentally ill in ancient Palestine, Greece, and Rome is that relatively little attention was devoted to the subject generally, and to the afflicted, specifically. The "causes" of madness, both natural and supernatural, were individualized in nature. They were located in forces that resided within the person of the mentally deranged, and these forces were apparently not subject to human mastery for the purpose of either preventive or therapeutic treatment. Because the causes of madness were considered to be so totally individual as compared to social, and because the care of the mentally ill was a private matter for the family, community responsibility or involvement with matters of madness was very rare.

Knowledge about mental illness or treatment of the mentally ill did not seem to change substantially through the Middle Ages and throughout the sixteenth century. Responsibility for the mentally disturbed still rested primarily with the family, although records indicate that some acute patients were admitted to general hospitals. There also are more recorded instances of public responsibility in cases of patients who were dangerous or without relatives, and there are municipality records which list maintenance costs for mentally disturbed persons without families who were placed in the home of some other person in the community.

The most interesting practice recorded in this historical period is that whereby communities took the mentally ill who were not native to the community and expelled them for return to their own towns.[5] Municipalities apparently undertook the costs of transporting the "foreigners," as well as payments to physicians who may have provided care for those deranged persons who were considered public responsibility. In some cases, the insane were not provided transportation but were simply given money and told to return to their own towns.

This practice seems to mark the beginning of formal expulsion of the insane from the community (although not the native insane), as well as acknowledgement of an extension of responsibility for the insane from the family to the community. Because the family group and the communal group were the two principal social anchors for people in this period, it is not surprising that expulsion of the mentally disturbed *began with strangers;* i.e., those from other towns. Yet once begun, the practice was eventually extended to members of the family or communal groups, as long as appropriate belief systems which justified the practice were developed.

THE BEGINNINGS OF CONFINEMENT

Foucault depicts the seventeenth and early eighteenth century in Europe as the period of the "great confinement." [6] It is a time in which the insane could be found in houses of confinement with the poor, unemployed, and criminals. Foucault marks the beginning of this period with a royal edict in 1656, in Paris, whch provided for an administrative reorganization of existing establishments and

[5] Ibid., p. 140.

[6] Michel Foucault, *Madness and Civilization* (New York: Vintage Books, 1973).

the creation of the *Hôpital Général.* All these establishments "were now assigned to the poor of Paris of both sexes, of all ages and from all localities, of whatever breeding and birth, in whatever state they may be, able-bodied or invalid, sick or convalescent, curable or incurable." [7]

The insane found themselves in special institutions not because of any special public concern with mental disorders, but because one aspect of the nature of madness—unemployment—coincided with the plight of the poor, unemployed, and other casualties of the economic crisis that affected Europe during this time. According to Foucault, it is clear, furthermore, that the *Hôpital Général* was not a medical establishment.

It is rather a sort of semijudicial structure, an administrative entity which, along with the already constituted powers, and outside of the courts, decides, judges, and executes. . . . A quasi-absolute sovereignty, jurisdiction without appeal, a writ of execution against which nothing can prevail—the *Hôpital Général* is a strange power that the king establishes between the police and the courts, at the limits of the law: a third order of repression.[8]

The practice of confining an undifferentiated mass of persons spread throughout Europe and served as one of the answers to the economic conditions that created thousands of persons "without resources, without social moorings, a class rejected or rendered mobile by economic developments." [9] Yet what this mass confinement of the insane along with assorted economic and social casualties did for the very first time was to focus public attention on the mentally deranged as a special problem. As Foucault points out in an important insight, when economic conditions changed, the unemployed and poor became a source of cheap manpower but the insane were left with the legacy of their former inmates' stigmas. Madness now ranked with other major problems, for the insane were now linked with poverty, inability to work, and inability to function as contributing members of society. This new problem status for madness was especially pronounced as new values were established which elevated the obligation to work to an ethical code, and which condemned idleness, sloth, and social uselessness.

Throughout most of the eighteenth century madmen shared con-

[7] Ibid., p. 39.
[8] Ibid., p. 40.
[9] Ibid., p. 48.

finement with criminals and shared their chains and dungeons as well. Contrary to popular belief, the separation of the mentally deranged from the criminal did not come from medical science, or from a new philosophy of care, or from humanitarian impulses. It came first, and with the loudest voice, according to Foucault, from the prisoners who were "indignant at being forced to live with madmen"; from the overseers whose function was to organize the work of prisoners and who complained that "the workshop is disturbed by the cries and the confusion of the insane"; and from those who saw the enforced association of the mad with those who were not mad as the ultimate in punishment and humiliation.

According to popular medical history, by the end of the eighteenth century the influence of such reformers as Tuke and Pinel resulted in the liberation of the insane, and brought forth "that happy age when madness was finally recognized and treated according to a truth to which we had too long remained blind." [10] Yet for Foucault, the "legends of Pinel and Tuke transmit mythical values" which obscure the actual consequences of their efforts to place the mentally ill in asylums. The isolation of madness and its location in a special institution had two profound effects: first, it made the physician the central and ultimate authority for the care and treatment of the mentally ill; and second, although it liberated the insane from physical constraints, it produced a total mastery of madness by making it an *object,* not only to be studied and controlled by others, but subject also to the madman's self-examination.

On the new role of the physician, Foucault states:

The work of Tuke and of Pinel, whose spirit and values are so different, meet in this transformation of the medical personage. The physician, as we have seen, played no part in the life of confinement. Now he becomes the essential figure of the asylum. He is in charge of entry. The ruling at the Retreat is precise: "On the admission of patients, the committee should, in general, require a certificate signed by a medical person. . . . It should also be stated whether the patient is afflicted with any complaint independent of insanity. It is also desirable that some account should be sent, how long the patient has been disordered; whether any, or what sort of medical means have been used." From the end of the eighteenth century, the medical certificate becomes almost obligatory for the confinement of madmen. But within the asylum itself, the doctor takes a preponderant place, insofar as he converts it into a medical space. However, and this is the essential point, the doctor's intervention is not made

[10] Ibid., p. 241.

by virtue of a medical skill or power that he possesses in himself and that would be justified by a body of objective knowledge.

It is thought that Tuke and Pinel opened the asylum to medical knowledge. They did not introduce science, but a personality, whose powers borrowed from science only their disguise, or at most their justification. These powers, by their nature, were of a moral and social order; they took root in the madman's minority status, in the insanity of his person, not of his mind. If the medical personage could isolate madness, it was not because he knew it, but because he mastered it.[11]

Finally, Foucault comments on the total mastery of madness achieved by its objectification:

We must therefore re-evaluate the meanings assigned to Tuke's work: liberation of the insane, abolition of constraint, constitution of a human milieu—these are only justifications. The real operations were different. In fact Tuke created an asylum where he substituted for the free terror of madness the stifling anguish of responsibility; fear no longer reigned on the other side of the prison gates, it now raged under the seals of conscience. Tuke now transferred the age-old terrors in which the insane had been trapped to the very heart of madness. The asylum no longer punished the madman's guilt, it is true; but it did more, it organized that guilt; it organized it for the madman as a consciousness of himself, and as a non-reciprocal relation to the keeper; it organized it for the man of reason as an awareness of the Other, a therapeutic intervention in the madman's existence. In other words, by this guilt the madman became an object of punishment always vulnerable to himself and to the Other; and, from the acknowledgement of his status as object, from the awareness of his guilt, the madman was to return to his awareness of himself as a free and responsible subject, and consequently to reason.[12]

After Tuke and Pinel, psychiatry became a special brand of medicine, and the doctor assumed magical qualities in relation to madness and in the organization of the asylum. What began at the end of the eighteenth century still finds expression in the rites of asylum life today.

GROWTH OF THE ASYLUM IN AMERICA: THE INSANE AS
CASUALTIES OF THE SOCIAL ORDER

The American experience in understanding and responding to mental illness parallels the European pattern described by Foucault

[11] Ibid., pp. 270, 271–72.

[12] Ibid., p. 247.

(1965) and Rosen (1968) in one important respect. In both societies the earliest recorded experiences indicate that insanity was dealt with as a part of normal, everyday life. The insane remained in families and, for the most part, were free to roam the streets and roads of town and countryside. Similarly, in both societies, the insane ultimately found themselves objectified; that is, they were viewed as special problems which required special care and treatment dispensed by specialists, in institutions constructed or organized with their special problems in mind.

Foucault's explanation of the transformation of madness from a state of inclusion to one of exclusion in European society is found in the role of Enlightenment thought which sought to bring all of social life, including madness, under the control of reason. The asylum became the place where the disordered mind could be mastered, and where reason would be brought to bear upon the forces of unreason.

In America, on the other hand, the early colonists assumed that the causes of insanity, like those of other diseases, were expressions of God's will. Conceptions of "treatment" of the insane (along with other deviants) consisted mainly of physical punishment, while care was mainly in the hands of families.[13] Those without families or with dangerous disorders found their way into the almshouse, which was used clearly as a last resort.

Throughout the eighteenth century the insane remained outside confinement in America. According to Rothman's study of the growth of the asylum in this country, before 1810 only a few states had institutions for the mentally ill. Yet by 1850 almost every Northeastern state legislature and many Midwest legislatures supported an asylum. By 1860, 28 of 33 states had public institutions for the insane, representing a striking growth in the use of asylums for the mentally ill. What was responsible for this movement to exclude the mentally ill from society? An advance of scientific knowledge about causes and treatments? A product of the growing power of medicine in general and psychiatry in particular? The adoption of European techniques and beliefs about mental illness? Rothman's answer to the question of why asylums flourished in the early nineteenth century in America contains two main parts. First, there

[13] David J. Rothman, *The Discovery of the Asylum* (Boston: Little, Brown and Co., 1971).

was particular belief in the causes of mental illness that gained a strong foothold in medical circles; and second, there was a belief that asylum life could serve as a therapeutic agent in the cure of mental disorders.

In the early eighteenth century the prevailing view of the cause of mental illness held by the medical community was that insanity was a disease of the brain which was characterized by organic lesions. Yet despite this, a segment of the medical community that was involved with mental disorder—medical superintendents— embraced a European idea that insanity was linked to civilization. For them, unrestrained ambition, the pursuit of success, and the increasing complexity of life became those features of society thought to be responsible for mental disorders. It was the American overzealous pursuit of wealth, power, and knowledge that was identified as the source of great personal stress. Not only were these goals pursued with great energy, but their attainment did not seem to satisfy. It seemed as if Americans were more interested in the frenzy of the race itself than in what the race for wealth, power, and knowledge would produce.

What the medical superintendents were doing was providing a critique of nineteenth-century America.[14] Their critique, more-over, was based upon the belief that the danger inherent in the new social order was the disruption of a stable, established order without the provision of new bases of stability and cohesion. As Rothman puts it:

Frightened by an awareness that the older order was passing and with little notion of what would replace it, they [medical superintendents] de-fined the realities about them as corrupting, provoking madness. The root of their difficulty was that they still adhered to the precepts of traditional social theory, to the ideas that they had inherited from the colonial period. By these standards, men were to take their rank in the hierarchy, know their place in society, and not compete to change positions. Children were to be content with their station, taking their father's position for their

---

[14] Although there is no such indication in the Rothman book, it is probable that the critique of American society made by the medical super-intendent was also influenced by the pastoralist writers who had developed their own criticism of technology and "progress" in the early nineteenth century. See, e.g., Leo Marx, *The Machine in the Garden: Technology and the Pastoral Ideal in America* (New York: Oxford University Press, 1964).

own. Politics and learning were to be the province of trained men, and ordinary citizens were to leave such matters to them. Family government was to instill order and discipline, and the community to support and reinforce its dictums. This was the prescription for a well-ordered society, one that would not generate epidemics of insanity.[15]

Even more dangerous, according to the medical superintendents, was the fact that the institutions that should be providing stability —the school, family, and church—were in fact not moderating the dangers inherent in the social order but adding to them. These institutions were alleged to encourage the excessive concern with success, and to praise as virtues excessive ambition and striving, and extensive time devoted to study.

But although the medical superintendents located the causes of mental illness in the social organization of society, they did not follow through and suggest that there should be changes in society. Instead, they proposed that the insane be placed in a setting that would eliminate the stress and strain of social life and provide them with the order and stability lacking in the larger society. Insane asylums were to be re-creations of the idealized colonial community and thereby provide mental patients with a therapeutic environment.

The basic principles underlying the structure of the asylum included the following:

1. The insane were to be removed from the community in order to be protected from the dangers of the community.

2. The asylum would be physically separate from the community, providing further protection from the dangers of the community as well as a peaceful rural landscape.

3. Families were discouraged from visiting with patients because they would disrupt hospital routine.

4. Asylum life should emphasize discipline, routine, neatness, fixed schedules, and work assignments for patients.

Rothman seems convinced that the medical superintendents' critique of the social order was primarily responsible for the governing principles that shaped asylum life. Yet it seems equally plausible that for the organization of the new asylum there lies a

---

[15] Rothman, *Discovery of the Asylum,* p. 127.

rationale that is less therapeutic in purpose, less patient-centered, and less influenced by the theories of the medical superintendents. The exclusion of patients from the community may have been a condition demanded by the community members themselves, and resulting in their support of asylums. The same may have been true for the determination of the location of asylums insofar as a combination of cheaper land and a desire to put the insane at some distance from the community were the determining factors. Finally, we may note here that many of the particular features of asylums which were advocated by the medical superintendents were ultimately discredited.

THE MODERN DEBATE: THE INSANE AS PATIENTS OR VICTIMS

The decline in the influence of medical superintendents took place as it became apparent that insanity was not being eradicated by the milieu therapy of the asylum. Pessimism about the ability to cure insanity through the environment of the asylum also served to discredit the general theory of causation put forward by the superintendents. If insanity was not caused by a sociey without order, discipline, and limits on ambition, where then were the causes to be found? The answer was provided quickly by medical practitioners who had always embraced a disease theory of mental illness but who had lacked the power to oppose the medical superintendents. Mental illness was once again viewed as a disease that had its origin and residence within the body of the insane, and could therefore be treated as any other disease of the body.

Since the turn of this century, then, conceptions of nature, cause, and treatment of mental illness have been products of a dominant framework that has been called the *medical model*. From the perspective of this model, mental illness is something that a person *has*, like cancer or heart disease. A person with mental illness exhibits peculiar, unusual, or problematic behavior which is related to some underlying cause that resides in the human organism. These behaviors are seen as "pathological symptoms" of a disease, and as such are subject to "diagnosis" and "treatment." The language and concepts of the medical model are unmistakably analogous to that of physical medicine, a fact which significantly influences the manner in which those afflicted with "mental disease" are treated.[16]

Strong support for the medical model of mental illness comes from those segments of the medical community who focus upon brain pathology as the basis of psychological symptoms, and those who stress the role of strictly medical treatment (as compared to "talk" therapies) to deal with behavior disorders.[17] Support has also come from members of the medical and mental health communities who, although they may not embrace a disease theory of mental illness, do subscribe to the view that mental illness is similar to physical illness. One consequence of the attempt to link mental and physical illness is that those concerned about mental illness are able to draw upon the resources and prestige of the medical community and its allies in their fight against mental disorder. A second consequence is an effort to remove the stigma of mental illness by giving it the same status as the common cold; the assumption is that people will lose their fear of mental illness and understand more about its treatment both in and out of hospitals, if it has the same status as a physical disease in the public's mind.[18]

The contribution of modern psychology to our understanding of mental illness has led to the emergence of a modification of the medical model into something called the *behavioral model*. This approach is based on a view that "the behaviors traditionally called abnormal are no different, either quantitatively or qualitatively, in their development and maintenance from other learned behaviors." [19] Abnormal behavior is simply viewed as an example of the application of the general behavioral model to the area of dysfunctional mental behavior. According to this view, deviant behavior is determined and maintained by environmental stimuli, and is the

---

[16] B. A. Maher, *Principles of Psychopathology: An Experimental Approach* (New York: McGraw-Hill, 1966).

[17] D. P. Ausubel, "Personality Disorder Is Disease," *American Psychologist*, 61 (February 1961), 69–74.

[18] Harrison M. Trice and Paul M. Roman, "Delabeling, Relabeling, and Alcoholics Anonymous," *Social Problems,* 17 (Spring 1970), pp. 538–46.

[19] L. P. Ullmann and L. Krasner, eds., *A Psychological Approach to Abnormal Behavior* (Englewood Cliffs, N.J.: Prentice-Hall, Inc., 1969), p. 1.

result of interaction with the social environment rather than a problem within the individual.

Both the medical and behavioral models of mental illness share a common focus upon the "individual system" as the entity to be diagnosed, studied, and treated. Dysfunctional mental behavior of individuals is observed, diagnosed, and categorized according to a classification system that is assumed to be descriptive of specific behaviors and useful for deciding upon a course of treatment. Whether the treatment method is behavior control, individual or group therapy, electroshock, or drugs, it is something that is done to individuals who are assumed to be sick and whose illness is to be alleviated by the treatment. The person who is identified as exhibiting dysfunctional mental behavior becomes, in the same sense as one with a physical illness, a *patient*.

In sharp contrast to this emphasis upon the individual as the carrier of a disease called mental illness is a relatively recent set of ideas, put forward mainly by sociologists, that has come to be called the *societal reaction model* of mental illness. The central feature of this emerging model is its shift of attention from individuals who are alleged to *have* a mental illness to the social groups that *create* mental illness by their application of social rules of conduct in judging what is or is not "normal" behavior. In this model, moreover, many of the behaviors which are viewed by current medical and lay conceptions as mental illness are not considered to be expressions of a disease inherent in the individual but, rather, behaviors that persons initially defined as sick develop to cope with their situation of having been so defined.

The distinction between the "problematic" behaviors that people may exhibit and the social groups that react to those behaviors is contained in Lemert's important separation of primary deviation from secondary deviation. As he states,

Primary deviation is assumed to arise in a wide variety of social, cultural, and psychological contexts, and at best has only marginal implications for the psychic structure of the individual. . . . Secondary deviation is deviant behavior, or social roles based upon it, which becomes a means of defense, attack or adaptation to the overt and covert problems created by the societal reaction to primary deviation.[20]

[20] Edwin Lemert, *Human Deviance, Social Problems and Social Control* (Englewood Cliffs, N.J.: Prentice-Hall, Inc., 1967), p. 17.

When applied to mental illness, the societal reaction perspective challenges the view that mental illness is the result of an underlying disease process or a set of learned pathological behaviors. Instead, it starts with the view that large segments of a population engage, at one time or another, in acts of primary deviance (i.e., rule breaking). This position is supported by studies which indicate that the presence of pathological symptoms which could warrant psychiatric hospitalization in *nonhospitalized* populations is substantial.[21] Scheff has noted that although some of these acts of primary deviation have well-established labels for the violations, "there is always a residue of the most diverse kinds of violations for which the culture provides no explicit label." [22] A combination of the above elements leads to a theory that views psychiatric symptoms as "labeled violations of social norms, and stable 'mental illness' to be a social role." [23] What differentiates rule breakers who do and those who do not become labeled as mentally ill is to be found in the characteristics of the social groups in which rule breakers are located, the power of the rule breakers, and the context and visibility of the rule breaking.

Thus, persons called mentally ill are not seen as patients, but as *victims*. They are victims of situational contingencies such that in one case an act of rule breaking will be transformed into a psychiatric symptom, whereas in another case the very same act may be ignored or dealt with in other than a psychiatric framework. They are victims of their vulnerable status in society which makes them less able to defend against more powerful family members or heavily credentialed experts whose job it is to pass judgment on the mental health of others. In addition, they are victims of their own humanness, which makes them responsive to the judgments of significant others whereby they take the views of others and internalize them as their own. In short, the social role of mental illness can be *created* by collective judgments, imposed upon those

[21] See, e.g., Leo Srole et al., *Mental Health in the Metropolis: The Midtown Manhattan Study*, Vol. 1 (New York: McGraw-Hill, 1962); and Benjamin Pasamanick, "A Survey of Mental Disease in an Urban Population, An Approach to Total Prevalence Rates," *Archives of General Psychiatry*, IV (August 1961), 151–55.

[22] Thomas Scheff, *Being Mentally Ill* (Chicago: Aldine, 1966), p. 34.

[23] Ibid., p. 25.

who are socially vulnerable, and voluntarily adopted by persons as a defensive strategy. The end result is not a patient with a disease, but a victim of a socially constructed reality.

MODELS OF MADNESS APPLIED TO THE MENTAL HOSPITAL

According to both the medical and behavioral models of mental illness, the reasons for hospitalizing someone judged to have a mental disorder are twofold. First, hospitalization removes the person from the demands and stresses of "normal" living. Obligations as a parent, wife, husband, worker, or citizen are suspended, thereby either eliminating a source of the illness or eliminating demands that might simply interfere with the therapeutic process. Second, it is assumed that the "treatment" to be applied to the "disease" must be repeated frequently, monitored frequently, evaluated for its effects, and modified or repeated in accordance with the results of evaluation.

Consistent with the societal reaction model, on the other hand, the main reasons for hospitalization are quite different. First, going to a mental hospital is the logical extension of the initial act of defining a person "outside" of the normal role boundaries of the family. Having approved of the family's right to define away the rights of its members, society accepts responsibility for total exclusion of the deviant from all aspects of "normal" social life. The second reason for hospitalization is that it represents an effort to stabilize the deviant role and reinforce the deviant identity of the victim. Thus, the mental hospital provides continuity for the deviant identification and identity that emerge in the primary group, and now are transferred to strangers who pass judgment on the normality of the committed person.

Assuming that the societal reaction model of mental illness is the most accurate explanation of the process that leads to hospitalization, release from the hospital requires the construction of a new social identity by the members of the patient's institutional "family," and the acceptance of the new identity by people outside the institution, who are now the strangers.

This takes us to the central theme of this book. It is our general view that madness is a communal affair. It is created, stabilized,

sustained, and discarded by groups of people and not by the person who is presumed to be ill. The mental hospital, however, does not officially embrace this view of madness. Rather, it represents the final culmination of a dualism in the idea of madness that can be traced throughout written histories of madness and which produces a series of incompatibilities and tensions that permeate the structure and operation of the mental hospital. This dualism is reflected in predominant medical and lay beliefs that madness is an individual affair, in that it is a disease that resides in the individual and requires as treatment something that is done to the individual. It is also reflected in the overpowering fact that entry or departure from a deviant social role, as with entry or release from the mental hospital, is in the hands of significant others whose decisions have only the most tenuous relation to the actual behaviors and "symptoms" of the victim.

This dualism in the conception of mental illness is not entirely unrecognized by those who say one thing but do another. Although it is not a matter that is openly and freely discussed by persons who participate in acts of commitment and hospital custody, it does touch the lives of all these people who in their private or intimate moments allow themselves to face up to things they suspect but repress in order to do what they do.

It is the staff of mental hospitals who carry the burden of this dualism. As persons who do the "dirty work" for a society that has chosen to exclude some of its members, they keep the "secret" of the dualism, and allay any suspicions that perhaps people in mental hospitals should not be there, and that what passes for diagnosis and treatment has little or nothing to do with getting well and being returned to society. The price that is paid by those who do the "dirty work" is to share some of the stigma of the patients with whom they work. It is as if society makes preparations to protect itself in the event that those who do the dirty work might one day expose the dualism in mental illness and the scientific and moral bankruptcy of the mental hospital.[24]

Thus, what we are suggesting is that doctors, nurses, and attend-

---

[24] For a discussion of the general problem of how society rewards selected members to carry out tasks that "good people" will not do but will support, see Everett C. Hughes, "Good People and Dirty Work," *Social Problems,* 10 (Summer 1964), 3–11.

ants in mental hospitals share a marginality and stigma with their patients that only further complicates the social order of the mental hospital. As any person who knows life in a mental hospital has probably observed, every so often a staff member will identify with the plight of a patient and view that patient as a victim of a family and the hospital. These occasional bonds that develop between staff and patients reflect the existence of the dual conceptions of mental illness and the recognition that the tension implied by the dualism does, in such individual cases, break through as a public matter.

The remainder of this book concerns the way in which life in the mental hospital for both patients and staff is affected by the communal nature of madness. Our observations on madness and the mental hospital are based upon a year of field work in a large state mental hospital in a Midwestern state. In order to protect the anonymity of persons involved in this study the hospital will be referred to as Riverview.

The year in the field was divided into four data collection stages. First was a period of general observation on the study ward and in other divisions of the hospital. Information on the social and medical history of each patient was extracted from hospital documents and recorded on precoded forms. The second period initiated the more systematic observation on the study ward. The observer divided his time on the ward between the nurses' office, the dayroom, and the smoking lounge. The observation periods in each location were varied by day and time. The patient-staff interaction reported in this book was charted in the nurses' office.

In the third period the sociometric data were collected, ward staff were interviewed, and systematic observation on the ward continued. The final stage was devoted to interviewing patients, systematic observation and verbatim recording of disposition staff meetings, and the distribution of a patient-centered questionnaire to the study ward attendants. Daily nursing notes and all charted information for each patient were recorded during the second and third phases of the study. At the close of the field work a mail questionnaire was sent to all doctors, nurses, attendants, and adjunct therapists in the hospital.

2

The Mental Hospital
As a People=Processing
Organization

Whether it is referred to as the "crazyhouse," the "state hospital," or by some idyllic-sounding euphemism such as "Longview" or "Briarcliff," the mental hospital is that social organization in which society places persons who are defined as being mentally ill. Official reports which describe the philosophy and goals of mental hospitals abound with statements which emphasize the treatment and rehabilitation of patients. Milieu therapy, reality therapy, attitude therapy, and behavior modification are identified as some of the treatment techniques which are being applied to disordered minds. Also stressed is a close working relationship between the hospital, the community, and the family which is designed to facilitate planning for a speedy discharge from the time a patient is admitted to a hospital. Such a consideration is reflected in the use of such organizational concepts as community liaisons, community reentry, family intervention, and community linkage. A final feature of official statements about philosophy and goals is the inevitable description of a new spirit of cooperation that has existed among hospital staff since the latest reorganization or since the introduction of some new administrative innovation. In this connection one is confronted with the ideas of team treatment, role blending, sensitivity groups, and management leadership.

Statements which describe the official goals of a mental hospital, or any organization for that matter, must be approached with caution, at least if one hopes to learn something about what actually goes on within that organization. Yet, despite the fact that one must be skeptical about official goals, it is very important to note the three features of a mental hospital that are being discussed in most statements about goals. First, there is the nature of the relationship that exists between the community and the hospital, and the steps that are being taken to ensure community cooperation and support. Second, there is the internal structure of the hospital in terms of the distribution of authority and responsibility. The third feature is the particular treatment technology that is being used to change patients, and hopefully, to effect their early release from the hospital.

Community-hospital relations, the internal structure of authority, and treatment technology are three central features of mental hospitals which one can use to facilitate understanding of the day-to-day life of patients and staff. These elements are in a continual state of change, reflecting shifting definitions of mental illness, the changing power of hospitals vis-à-vis the larger society, and the availability of new ideas about hospital organization and procedures. Thus, the mental hospital in its present form is an historically evolving social organization which is constantly attempting both to adapt and to control its internal and external environment. It reflects, moreover, imperfect evolution because the hospital contains elements which change at different paces, thereby producing an organization composed of "survivals" (i.e., things better suited to an earlier environment) and characterized by poor internal integration.

In this chapter, we examine some of the organizational problems that are peculiar to the mental hospital as a special type of organization that houses persons who have been rejected by society and that tries to return those persons to society. In addition, we consider some of the characteristics that mental hospitals share with other kinds of organizations. The general focus of the chapter is the influence of the external environment (i.e., society) and treatment technology upon the internal structure and processes of life inside the hospital.

ORGANIZATION AND ENVIRONMENT: THE QUESTION
OF POWER AND AUTONOMY

Every organization exists in a social and cultural environment that is more or less supportive of and conducive to the organization's existence. Social values, legal institutions, and the nature of the class structure create favorable or unfavorable climates for an organization, encourage or discourage people from working for or on behalf of the organization, and set limits upon the freedom with which the organization can pursue its goals.

Every organization, moreover, tries to exercise influence and control over its external environment in order to make easier the pursuit of its goals. In the most general sense, the organization-environment relationship concerns the nature of and control over the *inputs* an organization needs to carry on its work—money, raw materials, workers, physical facilities—and *outputs* of the organization. A favorable reception for an organization's output, whether it be consumer goods or "cured" ex-patients, provides an organization with a more favorable position for obtaining inputs for its continued existence.

The particular balance of power that exists between an organization and its environment is never really fixed, but is continually shifting in a manner that reflects an organization's relative success in adapting to its environment. As environment changes, so must an organization, or face the possibility of extinction. Take, for example, the Woman's Christian Temperance Union, an organization that "produced" a middle-class moral code.[1] The WCTU flourished as long as there was a natural market for its "output" or as long as it had the power to create such a market. When societal values changed, the WCTU lacked a marketable product and, hence, could not obtain sufficient resources (e.g., money, new members, support from other organizations) to stay in existence. In addition, the demise of the WCTU represents a case in which over-adaptation of an organization produces success in one period but total failure in another.

Looking at the mental hospital in historical perspective, one can see periods of relative autonomy and power of the hospital in relation to the larger society with respect to both inputs and outputs of the hospital. From the work of both Foucault[2] and Rothman,[3]

[1] Joseph Gusfield, "Social Structure and Moral Reform: A Study of the Woman's Christian Temperance Union," *American Journal of Sociology*, 61 (November 1955), 221–32.

[2] Michel Foucault, *Madness and Civilization* (New York: Vintage Books, 1973).

[3] David J. Rothman, *The Discovery of the Asylum* (Boston: Little, Brown and Co., 1971).

discussed in Chapter One, it is apparent that mental hospitals exercised considerable control over all their activities during the period in which they first emerged. In the United States in the early nineteenth century, medical superintendents (i.e., psychiatrists) apparently had sufficient influence with state legislatures to establish extensive autonomy over the design, cost, location, and internal structure of the new asylums. They also determined who entered hospitals as patients, who was allowed to visit patients, and who should be viewed as "cured." The superintendents were quite successful, apparently, in avoiding the involvement of civil authorities in the commitment process, and in convincing patients' families that the hospital alone should determine when patients should be released.[4]

Thus, in the early stage of the establishment of mental hospitals the professional staff exercised considerable power and autonomy in relation to the larger society. This period of power and autonomy, however, started to reverse itself in the latter half of the nineteenth century. The mental hospital and the medical superintendents were faced with two problems. The first came from state legislatures which, being much concerned about rising costs for the construction and maintenance of asylums, started to reduce appropriations. The second problem was criticism about the alleged success of the new institutions in "curing" the insane which came from medical professional groups outside the asylum (e.g., neurologists, research psychiatrists, psychiatrists in private practice).

Whatever were the causes of the decline in power and autonomy of the medical superintendents, it was manifested as a loss of control in the determination of who should enter the hospital. In many states, regulations on admissions were established whereby local officials and nonhospital professions were permitted to make such determinations. Superintendents were also denied the authority to determine the type of patients that would be admitted. Whereas in the past they were inclined to admit mainly those patients who had high potential for recovery, now they were forced to take indigent, chronic cases.

The loss of control over its "input" by the mental hospital, which began over a hundred years ago, continues to find expression in

4 Ibid., p. 143.

current hospital-society relationships. Across the fifty states, there can be found many different ways in which people become patients. There are emergency commitments made on the evaluation of a single physician; commitments made on the evaluation of two physicians; temporary or long-term commitments made by a judge; commitments made by a formally established county commission; and commitments made with and without court-appointed lawyers. These involuntary commitments have in common the fact that the decision is made by persons and bodies outside the hospital. Even the remaining major form of becoming a mental patient, "voluntary admission," leaves the hospital with little control insofar as they cannot hold the patient against his will without obtaining from an external body a regular, involuntary commitment.

Although there was a gradual erosion of hospital psychiatrists' control over who gets into a mental hospital, they continued to have considerable autonomy over the internal life of the hospital. Let us now turn to the matter of the social structure of the mental hospital itself.

HOSPITAL STRUCTURE

A visitor's first experience in a mental hospital leaves him with the impression of a well-organized bureaucratic structure. The superintendent sits at the apex of a structure that divides into clinical (i.e., medical) and business hierarchies. The medical side is further subdivided into functionally organized services and wards, each reflecting some aspect of a patient's career stage or particular medical needs. The positions within this general structure follow an almost classical caste-type structure. Caste lines are marked clearly and the symbols, speech patterns, and activities which serve to locate people within the structure are noticed quickly. Combined with clear lines of demarcation between positions in the hierarchy is the fact that there is little movement up or down the caste hierarchy; that is, there is no internal mobility.

Maintenance of the formal caste-like structure depends upon spatial separation, occupational separation, prescribed and proscribed activities for each stratum, rituals of avoidance, and shared symbolic representations of rank and status. Max Weber recognized these prerequisites for a caste system when he wrote that "complete 'fraternization' of castes has been and is impossible because it is one of the constitutive principles of the castes that there should be at least ritually irremediable barriers against complete commensalism among different castes." [5]

Herein lies one of the features of the hospital structure which is difficult to reconcile with stated therapeutic objectives. Although a rigid hospital structure is maintained through the above-stated mechanisms, treatment objectives are built upon premises of "fraternization" between hierarchical levels. The "team approach" in psychiatric treatment, for example, encourages interstatus contacts, open exchange of ideas and criticism, and free and unrestrained analysis of the behavior and motives of team members as they relate to patient care. Similarly, patients are usually thought to be well enough to leave the hospital when, in a sense, they "speak the language" of the superordinate groups. They adopt, so to speak, the staff values and norms which are transmitted through interpersonal relations. Yet this seeming contradiction in structure and goals is, in reality, a paradox only if one assumes that treatment and release of patients are serious goals of the hospital. This assumption will be examined more closely later in this chapter.

A second feature which has profound implications for the internal structure of the mental hospital is the fact that those who care for the mentally ill share some of the stigma that society places on patients. Early in this study the investigator had occasion to talk with people in the community nearest to a hospital about their awareness of the hospital's existence, its medical and economic role in the area, and its general influence on the attitudes of local residents. Oddly enough, rather than telling of fears of having "crazy people" so close, or expressing anticipated stereotyped views of the mentally ill, they offered views of the hospital staff which reflected a stigma that is reserved ordinarily for patients. Doctors were suspected of being "nuttier than the patients," or of being of questionable character or psychological health. For other staff, such as nurses and attendants, allegations were made that they were ex-patients themselves or had members of their family in the hospital at one time or another.

[5] Hans Gerth and C. Wright Mills, *Essays from Max Weber* (New York: Oxford University Press, 1958), p. 402.

The stigma attached by the community to staff personnel exists in the hospital itself. Hospital folklore and "in" jokes reveal numerous variations on the general theme that one often is not able to distinguish patients from staff. Much more important, however, is the fact that there is a clear indication of "marginality" among the medical staff especially. There are concrete examples of personal, career, and social marginality which help to fuel the stigma that is applied to the hospital staff. There is talk about problem drinkers, or career skidders who couldn't keep a private practice. In addition, there are the hospital doctors who have come from abroad to obtain psychiatric residencies in the United States. All of this adds to the view that many of the medical staff are doctors who are marginal within their own profession and this serves to reinforce, if not to cause, the stereotypes held both by members of the community and by the hospital.

If it is true that the "keepers" share a stigma with their "charges" we know something about the source of some of the problems concerning the structure of authority in the hospital and its ability to function either bureaucratically or therapeutically. In addition, we know something about the role of the mental hospital in our society, another point to which we shall return very shortly.

A third aspect of the mental hospital of import for its internal structure is the fact that its "raw materials" are humans, who must actively participate in their own transformation and in the general support activities of the hospital.[6] If one considers the patient as a client of an organization in the most general sense, one has the relatively rare situation wherein the client is a full-time member of the organization. On occasion a particular client functions outside the client role (i.e., a patient) and becomes a member of the occupational structure of the organization, carrying out essential activities regarding laundry, food, clothing, maintenance, and housekeeping.

The situation wherein a client is a full-time member of an organization can result in a variety of control and authority problems; that is, problems which result from a patient's access to knowledge of hospital affairs to which staff members only are supposed to be

[6] For a general theoretical treatment of alternative orientations of organization members or clients, see Amitai Etzioni, *A Comparative Analysis of Complex Organizations* (New York: The Free Press of Glencoe, Inc., 1961), Chapters 1–3.

privy. In addition, as a full-time working member of the hospital organization, the client plays a dual role which has considerable built-in personal as well as organizational tension. It is difficult to be a subordinate, passive person who is assumed to be experiencing problems of living, impaired reason, and irresponsibility while holding a full-time "job" in the hospital kitchen or laundry that a "normal" person would have to be hired to do otherwise.

To be a mental patient also requires one to participate actively in one's own transformation from "sick" raw material to "well" finished product. The degree of participation that is required is more than simple cooperation with the people and processes applied in order to produce a change, as would be the case for a patient in a general hospital. The mental patient must be active to the extent of negotiating with people in the environment and creating a new definition of reality for and about himself. A patient in such a situation will find incompatible demands between the needs of an orderly, bureaucratic, caste-like structure and an active, potent behavior of a "normal" person.

TECHNOLOGY AND TREATMENT GOALS

Organizational theory provides a general hypothesis to explain why mental hospitals have little power in their relations with society, and why hospital structure, staff, and goals seem to be so unsuccessful in the treatment of mental illness. The general view is that the nature of the technology an organization uses to transform raw material has a substantial influence on the internal structure of that organization.[7] Perrow has applied this point of view most convincingly to an examination of existing technology, structure, and goals of the mental hospital.[8]

Perrow's basic position is that the structure and goals of a mental hospital cannot be changed successfully without a change in technology. He maintains, furthermore, that hospitals do not have a

[7] James D. Thompson and Fred L. Bates, "Technology, Organization, and Administration," *Administrative Science Quarterly*, 2 (1957), 325–43.

[8] Charles Perrow, "Hospitals: Technology, Structure, and Goals," in James G. March, ed., *Handbook of Organizations* (Chicago: Rand McNally & Co., 1965), pp. 910–71.

treatment technology that is suited for the large number of patients they hold. "Milieu therapy," which is often described by hospital staff as a treatment technique, is, according to Perrow, not a new technology but a humanizing influence. His position is stated clearly in an analysis of mental hospitals' greater emphasis on custodial goals rather than treatment goals.

Hospitals are said to have "displaced" the treatment goal in favor of custody. It is more appropriate to say that the goal of "treatment" is of symbolic value only, and the real, operative goal is custody and minimal care.[9]

An extension of the logic of the technology hypothesis to several of the features of the mental hospital which were discussed earlier in this chapter leads to the following interpretations. First, the limited power and autonomy of the hospital to determine its "inputs" (i.e., patients) is a result of its inability to demonstrate to society that it can "cure" mental patients. Power and autonomy flow from ability to produce a marketable product, in this case a "cured" patient whom society is once again willing to accept. When and if the hospital has a technology that produces such a product, it will have more influence than it now commands. Second, the stigma attached to hospital medical staff and their marginal status within both the hospital and their profession are also results of their inability to demonstrate competence and expertise in their work.

There is much to be said for the technology hypothesis as a way of understanding the mental hospital. I believe it is especially powerful for furthering the understanding of the internal structure of the hospital in terms of authority and power relations. Yet one must be careful not to overstate the influence of technology or to assume that the utility of technology is inherent in it, and thereby cannot help being recognized as existing. Prevailing values, interests, and power will *interpret* new technology and help to shape claims regarding its worth. Thus, it is possible that hospital psychiatrists who have societal regard *because they are doing valued work* would also have the influence to shape a belief that "milieu therapy" is effective.

This brings us to our central criticism of the technology hypothe-

[9] Ibid., p. 926.

sis and the basis for an alternative view of mental hospitals which will follow. When it is argued that an effective treatment technology is needed to produce changes in hospital structure and goals, the basic assumption is that patients in the hospital do have something called a mental illness and do require a specific treatment in order to get "better." In short, it is assumed that the medical model of mental illness, as discussed in Chapter One, contains the best explanation of why people are committed to mental hospitals. If, however, hospital commitment takes place for the reasons described in the societal reaction model, the presence or absence of an effective treatment technology will have little connection with the treatment received by patients or their chances for getting out of a hospital. In other words, if one is in the hospital because one has been rejected by society, the purpose of the mental hospital is to make sure that one doesn't return to society. This view of the mental hospital is developed next.

PATIENTS AS VICTIMS AND THE HOSPITAL AS A SYSTEM OF JUSTIFICATION

One cannot begin to understand the way a mental hospital is organized and the way it operates without an understanding of why people are placed in hospitals in the first place. We, therefore, take here as our point of departure the societal reaction model of mental illness, which views patients as victims of the social networks in which they are embedded. They are victims of families and communities who can no longer tolerate rule-breaking and problematic behavior. They are victims of poverty, powerlessness, and discrimination and the resulting individual-psychological explanations for their plight as people with a mental illness. They, moreover, are often willing victims insofar as they accept and adopt the roles of madness in order to "solve" the problems of living which they are experiencing. In short, they are not in the hospital because they are mad, but because they have been rejected by society and have no suitable place in it.

The view of patients as victims is a very painful idea to accept by the individuals and families who are involved in putting someone in a mental hospital, and by the society that allows commitment to take place. In fact, the idea is so painful that individual and collective defense mechanisms develop to protect against the idea. An individual defense mechanism is the belief that mental illness is a disease, which makes it less difficult to put a family member in a mental hospital. A collective defense mechanism is the existence of a mental hospital as a social organization, which reinforces the belief in mental illness and espouses the noble goal of treatment and return of people to society, but which, in fact, functions in large part as a dumping ground for societal rejects.

This general perspective on mental illness and mental hospitals helps to illuminate some of the specific features of hospital organization which were discussed earlier in this chapter and in Chapter One. A discussion of these features follows.

The Establishment of Mental Hospitals. The question of when and why mental hospitals were established in the United States was discussed in Chapter One. It will be remembered that Rothman[10] put forward the hypothesis that the conditions conducive to the establishment of mental hospitals could be traced to a cluster of *ideas* about how the disorganization of traditional institutions was the cause of mental illness, and how the order, regularity, and discipline of the asylum could provide a cure for mental disorders.

There is no doubt about the existence of such ideas during the time that the mental hospital was becoming an established institution. What can be disputed, however, is whether or not such ideas were causal conditions for the creation of mental hospitals rather than a set of ideological justifications for a social organization that was brought into being for quite different reasons. What, then, would be the causal factors? Let us consider the following alternate hypotheses which would be consistent with our view of patients as victims and rejects.

The period during which mental hospitals became established institutions, 1830 to 1860, was characterized by certain social conditions that could have created a segment of the population who were without social moorings and were especially vulnerable to being victimized. By 1850, a pattern of urban settlement began to

[10] Rothman, *Discovery of the Asylum.*

be established, especially in the Northeastern states.[11] In addition, at about the same time almost one-half of the labor force was employed outside agriculture, a condition that coincided with a rural to urban area population shift and created a population of "new" people in unfamiliar surroundings who lacked supportive social ties. In fact, in 1850, 24 percent of the native-born population were residents of a state other than the one in which they were born, the highest such percentage over a 100-year period.[12]

Perhaps most significant, however, is the fact that the period of growth of asylums coincided with a period of substantial increases in immigration to the United States. The decade 1820 to 1830 brought 151,824 immigrants. From 1831 to 1840, the number increased to 599,125. For 1841 to 1850, the figure is 1,713,251, and for 1851 to 1860, the number increased to 2½ million.[13] In addition, there is some evidence that immigrants were substantially over-represented among patients in mental hospitals. Worcester State Hospital, for example, established in Massachusetts in 1833, had by 1851 over 40 percent foreign-born patients.[14]

Thus, it is suggested that the asylum may have emerged in America in order to deal with casualties of a changing social order in much the same way that the period of the "great confinement" in France, which marked the beginning of the institutionalization of the mentally ill there, was carried out to cope with the casualties of economic depression. In each case, it is the poor, the powerless, the socially vulnerable who are judged to be problems by families and communities, and whose problems are described as a form of illness which requires that they be expelled from normal social life.

Internal Structure: Authority of Physicians. If the societal reaction perspective has any validity as an explanation of why people enter mental hospitals, then it follows that those who are selected to care for the mentally ill are both personally oriented and pro-

[11] Noel P. Gist and Sylvia F. Fava, *Urban Society* (New York: Thomas Y. Crowell Co., 1964), p. 50.

[12] *Statistical Abstracts of the United States* (Washington, D.C.: U.S. Government Printing Office, 1952), p. 41.

[13] *Statistical Abstracts of the United States*, 1961, p. 92.

[14] Rothman, *Discovery of the Asylum*, p. 273.

fessionally equipped to provide long-term care for custody rather than treatment for release. Thus, the gravitation of personally and professionally marginal physicians to positions of authority in mental hospitals serves an important dual function. First, the high social standing of the position of doctor serves to rationalize and justify otherwise painful decisions which are made by families who commit "loved ones." After all, they could say, "It's not as if we are sending him to a prison or a detention center; he is going to a medical facility where humane care and treatment are available."

Second, because the physicians are neither personally nor professionally equipped to provide treatment, and because the hospital's patient-physician ratio makes treatment impossible even if physicians were equipped to provide it, physicians serve as convenient targets for complaints of "incompetence" at such times when society's "conscience" is stirred about the plight of the mentally ill.

The combination of marginality and stigma makes the physician especially vulnerable to challenges to his authority. He faces the classic dilemma inherent in bureaucratic authority in which the holder of a position of authority does not or cannot validate positional authority with demonstrated expertise. Authority based upon position alone is unstable and will be eroded eventually in relations with subordinates.[15]

Treatment Technologies. Most large state mental hospitals have experienced similar patterns of experimentation and use of various treatment technologies. Early use of physical techniques including psychosurgery, insulin and electroshock, hydrotherapy, and drugs seems to follow a sequence of early optimism about the effectiveness of the procedure, followed by doubts and eventual cessation of use entirely. Some of the physical techniques continue to be used. During the year in which Riverview was studied by this writer, the total patient population was approximately 2,400 persons. A total of 751 patients received 4,851 treatments of electroconvulsive therapy, and 131 patients received 2,337 treatments of hydrotherapy

---

[15] Concerning this general problem in organizations, see William M. Evan and Morris Zelditch, Jr., "A Laboratory Experiment on Bureaucratic Authority," *American Sociological Review,* 26 (December 1961), pp. 883–93.

for a total of 4,724 hours. During the same year, a total of 368 hours of individual and group psychotherapy took place, with a maximum of 45 hours in any single month. There is no record of the exact number of patients involved in such "talk therapies" but it is clear that the number is very small.

Psychopharmacological drugs are used extensively in the hospital and, like hydrotherapy, are viewed officially as parts of an overall therapeutic prescription for a patient rather than as total treatment techniques.

Following the use of physical technologies and "talk therapies," both of which were generally ineffective or impractical, came a large-scale effort to alter organizational arrangements in hospitals under the heading of "milieu therapy." Efforts to change the organizational structure concentrated upon increasing the communication between patients and staff in ways that would create consistent and reinforcing relationships among these groups. A part of milieu therapy involved the creation of "therapeutic teams" which shared total responsibility for all aspects of custody and treatment for a specific number of hospital patients. The "teams" emphasized open communication and shared authority among its members and more humane, equalitarian relations with patients.

The most recent organizational innovation that falls under the heading of milieu therapy is the transformation of the total hospital from a highly centralized, authoritarian structure to a decentralized structure with about eight to twelve treatment units which serve specific geographical areas (i.e., counties) in the state. Each unit has its own authority structure which is separate from the central administrator (i.e., superintendent) and which is based upon broadly representative committees rather than a single centralized authority. The "unit system" can be seen as an extension of therapeutic teams to the total hospital structure.

The "unit system" allows each team to develop its own programs and treatment strategies. The territorial basis for the unit encourages the development of more ties with and information about patients' families, community agencies, and community public services. All these efforts are aimed at the patient's planning discharge from the very time he is admitted.

As was pointed out earlier in this chapter, Perrow's analysis of mental hospitals criticized such efforts of "milieu therapy" as being simply examples of humane treatment rather than an effective treatment technology. We feel, however, that to view the efforts of milieu therapy within the narrow framework of physical technologies which are designed to treat a disease that resides in the individual is to misunderstand their significance. The unit system, for example, has two main consequences. First, it represents an effort to wrest control from physicians within the hospital's authority structure and to give expanded power to social workers, psychologists, and those nursing-attendant staff who have a strong interest in community mental health. The community mental health perspective is less inclined to view help for a mental patient as a matter of applying an effective technology to a disease that resides in an individual, and more likely to view treatment as a matter of keeping a patient in the family and in the community by working with families and community agencies to provide support for the patient. In short, the struggle for control is seen as a struggle between those whose professional work is guided by the medical model and those whose work is guided by the societal reaction model.

The second consequence of the unit system is that it attempts to establish for the hospital the power to determine who becomes a patient through ties to community mental health facilities, and it maintains the receptivity of families to accept ex-patients through its effort to ensure that families continue to accept responsibility for any of their members who are in the hospital.

Thus, attempts at "milieu therapy" might be very effective if they are guided by an understanding of the societal reaction model, and if they do enable the hospital to exercise more control over who enters it and over families to accept former patients as family members once again. If nothing else, milieu therapy efforts such as the unit system may discourage families, community physicians, and local legal authorities from moving too quickly to label people as mentally ill and to seek their hospitalization.

What is suggested in this section, then, is that the mental hospital functions primarily as a system of justification for a commitment process which cannot openly be admitted to be what it is; namely, a victimization process. The official purposes and ideology of the hospital are consonant with the medical model of mental illness. People who have a disease called mental illness are sent to a medical facility for diagnosis, treatment, and rehabilitation. The actual goals and activities of the hospital, however, are consonant with the view that patients are victims who have been expelled from their homes and communities in much the same way that madmen were expelled from their villages in the Middle Ages. Given the way in which the hospital is funded, staffed, and organized, it cannot help preventing patient victims from returning to society unless someone wants them.

REMAINDER OF THE BOOK

The remaining chapters of this book are devoted to more detailed examinations of a number of themes, hypotheses, and processes which have been touched upon in the initial two chapters. Chapter Three describes everyday activities in the hospital and the kind of adaptations made by patients to the exigencies of hospital life. Contrary to official ideology, everyday life in the hospital is not free of the tensions and demands that one faces outside the hospital and this vitiates one of the reasons why hospitalization is supposed to be helpful.

Chapters Four and Five analyze the quality and quantity of patient-staff, patient-patient, and staff-staff interaction. These relationships are related to the hospital's caste system and to the absence of opportunities for mobility for lower staff and patients. In addition, these relationships give patients the opportunity to "construct" new social roles for themselves and to use the organization to their own advantage.

Chapter Six focuses upon the patient belief system concerning ways to get out of the hospital. The breakdown of the patients' "release ideology" is related to the occurrence of a collective disturbance in the hospital. The relevance of "magical" belief systems in the mental hospital and other total institutions is examined.

Chapter Seven concerns one of the most significant events in the life of a patient. "Going to staff" is the situation in which decisions about discharge and long-term leave are made. Verbatim notes of discharge decisions are analyzed and several hypotheses about the type of patients and conditions most likely to lead to a discharge are offered.

The final chapter of the book presents some general conclusions about the relationship between madness and society and about the place of the mental hospital in this relationship.

II

THE NORMALITY
OF ORGANIZED MADNESS

3

Everyday Life:
Routines and Adaptations

This chapter provides a general picture of the formal structure of Riverview Hospital in terms of treatment sections, ward arrangements, staff locations, and the like. We shall also describe the kind of adaptations made by patients in order to survive in the hospital. A combination of daily routines and adaptations indicates that hospital life is anything but free of the tensions and anxieties that the patient is being protected from by hospitalization. In a sense, we hope to provide a base line from which the reader can view our later discussions of the hospital social structure.

The most pronounced organizational division of Riverview is to be found in its three separate treatment services. The three services represent a time sequence of movement through the hospital from the time a patient enters the hospital. Each service represents an implicit set of ideas regarding patient prognosis and the allocation of staff time and resources. The three services are:

Acute Intensive Treatment Service (AIT): The more acute, younger admissions, for whom discharge can more legitimately be expected within six months, will be retained on this service for more intensive treatment. The treatment includes all therapeutic services with the objective of having these patients discharged directly from this service, rather than at any time being exposed to the areas of the hospital caring for longer-term cases.

Intermediate Treatment Service (IT): This service, in contrast to AIT, seeks a more diversified, overall treatment program which will lead to an accelerated convalescent leave program.

Continued Treatment Service (CT):   Rehabilitative efforts in this service are directed primarily toward convalescent leaves to families, nursing homes, and to county homes. It focuses on those geriatric and/or better stabilized, chronically ill, older patients who can be cared for outside a situation of controlled care.

Within the three services are a total of twenty-four wards: six AIT; eight IT; and ten CT wards. This includes both male and female wards, open and closed wards. There are in addition two other services, the Tuberculosis Service and the Medical and Surgical Service. Essentially, these operate within a nonpsychiatric framework in terms of their work with patients.

Riverview, along with most large state hospitals, is faced with the problem of an inadequate number of professional personnel to handle the expanding patient population. Ward physicians find themselves responsible for the care of anywhere from fifty to four hundred patients on AIT and IT services. Physicians on CT wards often find the burden even greater. Table 3-1 provides a picture of the patient-staff distribution.

Comparing Riverview to the available figures of other state hospitals, the understaffing at professional levels is not atypical. From these figures one could easily deduce the nature of the psychiatric treatment possible under such conditions. For the acutely ill, tranquilizing and mood-elevating drugs are in extensive use; electroconvulsive therapy is also used in selected cases. For the chronically ill, remotivation and resocialization techniques are implemented through the various activity therapies. Population pressures have been translated into greater intellectual support for the merits of group psychotherapy rather than individual psychotherapy. The main development, however, has been in the extensive use of drugs, which are relatively easier to dispense to large numbers of patients.

Ward X

During the one-year study of Riverview, one ward was selected for more intensive study. The ward selected was a female open ward located in the Intermediate Treatment Service. It is housed in a rectangular two-story building in which it occupies the entire lower level. The physical layout of Ward X is represented in Figure 3-1.

A total of eighteen bedrooms is available for the patients. The number of patients per room varies from two to seven. For the most part the rooms are standardized, containing the beds, dressers, and an occasional straight-back chair or rocker. A few rooms exhibit re-

TABLE 3-1

DISTRIBUTION OF STAFF PERSONNEL AND
PATIENT-STAFF RATIOS AT RIVERVIEW

Position	Number	%	Patient-Staff Ratio*
Psychiatric Physician	9	1.2	255.6
Registered Nurse	28	3.7	82.1
Psychologist	6	.8	383.3
Psychiatric Social Worker	7	.9	328.6
Adjunctive Therapist**	11	1.4	209.1
Attendant	402	53.2	5.7
Other Full-Time Employees***	293	38.8	7.8
Totals	756	100.0	3.0

* This ratio is based upon a patient population of 2,300. Patients on leave, work placements, etc. were excluded.
** Work therapists, recreation workers, and occupational therapists are included here.
*** Included here are clerical staff, maintenance personnel, and dietary personnel.

ligious pictures on the walls, or magazine cutouts of flowers or animals. The doors to each room have a double narrow window space running half the length of the door. There is no glass in the panes, and the inner portions of the rooms are easily accessible to the glance of anyone walking down the hall. Rooms are generally empty during the day. Many are kept locked to keep patients from spending their entire day in their room. Access to one's room or bed, during the day, therefore becomes a privilege to be earned.

The very large dayroom is the center of activity on the ward. In the center section of the room are rows of about fifty comfortable

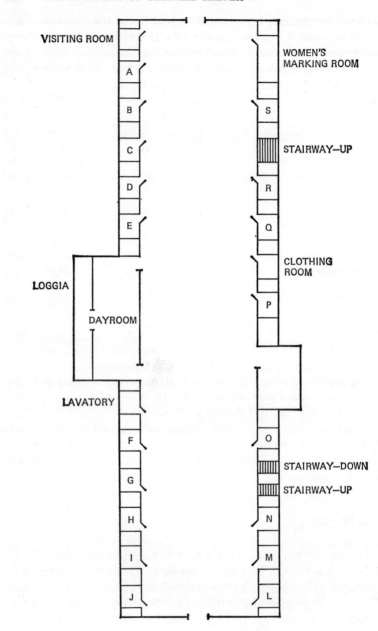

chairs. They are arranged in a classroom fashion in front of a television set. The TV set is in front of a large unused fireplace, over which hangs a picture of an early American president. Two of the walls are lined with what could be called daybeds. Patients who cannot lie in their rooms spend their time on the daybeds.

The rear wall of the dayroom, opposite the TV wall, has a double-door entrance to the loggia or sunroom. This is where all the smoking and talking takes place. It is the only place on the ward where smoking is permitted. The orderliness of the physical arrangements on the ward is quite pronounced. Chairs, couches, beds, and dressers can be found in the same positions on the ward for indefinite periods of time.

The nurses' office is opposite one of the entrances to the dayroom. The office has a "dutch door" which allows patients to talk to staff without entering the office. Inside the office are a desk, several chairs, an open cabinet containing patient charts, two closed and locked cabinets containing medications and drugs, a refrigerator, and the staff lavatory.

In the hall directly alongside the nurses' office is the "signout" desk. When patients leave the ward, they indicate where they are going and the time of departure. Upon returning, they again indicate the time and sign in. On the desk is a suggestion box with a padlock on it. Above the desk is a bulletin board.

The entire physical environment of the ward is lacking in potential "usefulness" to the patients. In other words, one cannot manipulate the physical environment for his own purposes: to seek more privacy, to seek individual expression through it, or to use it as a refuge. The ward belongs to everyone and to no one. As a result it has a certain "flatness" that belies the fact that people live there.

WARD X STAFF

Staff personnel with direct responsibilities on the ward are the ward doctor, ward nurse, ward attendants, social worker, and work therapist. The attendants alone are occupied by full-time duties on Ward X. All other personnel divide their time over a number of wards.

The ward physician generally makes at least one regular visit to the ward during the week. On the average he probably spends one and one-half hours on the ward each weekday. At this time he sees patients who have made requests to see him, handling such problems as plans for going out of the hospital on work placement, or advice concerning a love affair with a male patient. In many respects, the ward physician operates as a general problem solver. A large part of his time on the ward is spent writing or signing medical orders, ironing out administrative problems, and discussing with other staff the latest problem patient on the ward. Every other week, the physician conducts "ward rounds." At this time all the patients gather in the dayroom while the physician, followed by other ward staff, walks from patient to patient inquiring about their general state, and seeking questions. This procedure, again, is a response to the understaffing problem in that it provides some contact with the ward physician for all patients.

A major task of the ward physician is coordinating the activities of all other ward personnel. At times it is hard to tell who looks forward to the physician's daily visits more, the patients or the staff. In many ways, he must keep peace between the ward staff members and between staff and patients. Often, as a dispute mediator, he is urged to take sides to determine who is "right," the patient or the attendant, the social worker or the nurse, and so on. His general position on the ward depends, in part, on his handling of such situations.

The ward nurse, who also has responsibilities on other wards, will be found on Ward X three or four times a day for relatively short periods of time. She is the immediate supervisor of attendants, and operates as the conveyor of information, requests, and complaints from the attendants to appropriate persons. In many ways, the nurse is set up as a key figure for maintaining the locus of control for a greatly outnumbered professional staff. Attendants are repeatedly reminded not to "go over the head" of the ward nurse, but to work through her.

The nurse's duties on the ward are less clearly defined than those of any other person in the hospital. Her training as a medical nurse is only rarely called into play. As a psychiatric nurse, her particular skills and knowledge may extend beyond those of the ward attendant, but they have no opportunity for expression. Between the doctor, nurse, and attendant, the nurse has by far the least amount of contact with the patients. The reasons for this are not entirely formal either, for, in a sense, when the patient parcels out his time for contacts with ward personnel, contacts with the nurse usually provide the smallest margin of reward in terms of favors and extra privileges.

Attendants are the low people on the staff totem pole. They are responsible for housekeeping functions, sanitation, personal hygiene of patients, keeping records and preparing routine reports, and maintaining order on the ward. All these aspects of their work are deemphasized in favor of their contacts with patients.[1] Attendants have more contact and more *raw* knowledge of the patients than anyone else in the hospital. It is interesting in this connection to note that traditionally the hospital has not encouraged attendants, and in some instances did not allow them to read the master folders of patients on their ward. It is not hard to imagine the implications of a situation in which the person of lowest status has the most knowledge concerning the patients.

Much of the attendants' time is spent on dispensing and charting medications. Little opportunity is available for writing notes about patients' behavior on charts, except in extreme situations such as a fight, a combative patient, or very pronounced shifts in behavior. Lack of time is the standard cry of the attendants. These complaints generally dwell on the lack of time to spend with patients, and the lack of understanding by the administration of the important therapeutic function of the attendants.

The social worker and work therapist are rarely on the ward. The former will see patients in his office concerning contacts with the family, seeking work placements or family care placements for the patients, and working out plans for leaves. On occasion the social worker will establish individual therapy sessions for certain patients. The work therapist is primarily concerned with locating patients in various work assignments in the hospital. He screens the complaints

[1] For information on this particular point, see Richard L. Simpson and Ida Harper Simpson, "The Psychiatric Attendant: Development of an Occupational Self-Image in a Low-Status Occupation," *American Sociological Review*, 24 (June 1959), 389–92.

of working patients and the complaints of the patients' work supervisors.

THE PATIENTS

Ward X, operating at full capacity, houses fifty patients. Because
of some turnover in patients, we will include fifty-four patients in
our description of the patients on Ward X. Our purpose here is not
to discuss the patients in detail, but to provide some general description of the composition of the patient group by such characteristics
as age, diagnosis, and education.

From Table 3-2 we can see the variations in age, education, and

TABLE 3-2

DISTRIBUTION OF SELECTED CHARACTERISTICS OF PATIENTS ON WARD X

Age	No.	%	Education	No.	%	Diagnosis	No.	%
20–29	7	13.0	8th grade or less	20	37.0	Schizophrenic,		
30–39	12	22.2	Some high school	14	25.9	Paranoid Type	9	16.7
40–49	15	27.8	Completed			Schizophrenic,		
			high school	15	27.8	Catatonic Type	13	24.1
50–59	10	18.5	Some college	2	3.7	Schizophrenic,		
60–69	7	13.0	Completed college	2	3.7	Other	19	35.2
70+	3	5.5	Business of nursing			Manic-Depressive	3	5.5
			school	1	1.8	Mental Deficiency	4	7.4
						Organic, Other	3	5.5
						Psychoneurotic	3	5.5
Totals	54	100.0		54	99.9		54	99.9

diagnosis on Ward X. The age distribution reveals a median age of
approximately 45 years, with an overall diversity in the number of
relatively old and relatively young patients. Educational background, on the other hand, is primarily confined to the less than
high school categories, with relatively few patients having more
than a high school education.

In terms of diagnosis, the ward is made up primarily of patients
classified under some type of schizophrenic reaction. We have maintained the distinction between "paranoid type" and "catatonic type"

not because they may indicate some well-established psychiatric meaning, but because they have symbolic significance in the language of the hospital culture. For example, a patient may be spoken of as a "paranoid schiz" or a "catatonic schiz," but very rarely is he tagged as a "chronic undifferentiated schiz" in the everyday language on the ward. Aside from the schizophrenic category, there are only several patients in each of the other diagnostic groups.

A TYPICAL DAY ON THE WARD

Let us try to fill out this bare framework with a fuller description of routine events on the ward during an average day.

5:30 A.M. Patients working the dining rooms are awakened. They quietly go about dressing and using the lavatory and leave the ward by 6:00 A.M.

6:15 A.M. The night attendant, Mrs. Calen, turns on the lights and awakens all patients. Some patients are already awake, others rise quickly. Mrs. Calen is having her usual time getting Joan B. out of bed. Joan runs the gamut of complaints from "not feeling good" to "I'm too nervous to go to work today." Mrs. Calen counters each complaint with, "You'll feel better once you get up" or "Have some breakfast first and then see how you feel." Joan knows that once she concedes to an alternative her battle is lost. Down the hall some-one shouts, "Goddammit Celine, turn off that radio. It's getting so you can't hear yourself think around here." The patients' lavatory is used on a first-come first-serve basis. Minor encounters arise concerning who left the messy sink, or who left wet stockings to dry where they shouldn't be.

6:30 A.M. Medication is dispensed at the nurses' office by Mrs. Calen. Medication for each patient has been "set up" beforehand and is quickly and easily taken. Certain patients are asked to open their mouths in order to see if the pill is being held under the tongue, to be spit out later. Most patients go out to the loggia after medication for their first cigarette of the day.

6:45 A.M. Patients return to their rooms to make beds and straighten up. Very often patients debate the questions of who swept last, or who made the beds last.

7:15 A.M. The patients leave for breakfast in a group accompanied by Mrs. Calen. They return to the ward separately for roll call. The doors to the ward are left unlocked after breakfast.

7:45 A.M. The day-shift attendants, Mrs. Talbot and Mrs. Bender, come on the ward. Patients gather in the dayroom. Mrs. Calen calls the roll while Mrs. Talbot, the charge attendant, checks the signout book for patients who have left the ward early. Announcements are made by Nora P., ward president and representative to inter-ward council, that the inter-ward council meeting is being held on Ward L, and all are welcome to attend.

Occasional bickering takes place during the roll call: Betty L. makes a comment about Lizzie S.'s sloppy table manners at breakfast; several patients do a "cry baby" mimicking of the way Celine B. says, "Here, Mrs. Talbot"; Julia T. tells her latest psychiatrist joke, receiving open laughter from the patients, and a combination of censure and support from Mrs. Talbot, who says "Now, Julia."

8:00 A.M. Patients with regular work assignments sign out for work; others with ward work assignments go about their duties. Betty L., in charge of cleaning the dayroom, hall, and nurses' office, proceeds to order patients in and out of various areas she is working in.

Other patients without formal duties sign out to the library or the canteen.

After cleaning is over, several patients return to the ward and gather out on the loggia.

DOROTHY   I heard where there's a carnival coming to the hospital this summer.

(*No one responds to her comment.*)

LIZZIE   Hey, Nellie, do you want to walk down to the canteen with me?

NELLIE   No, I'm too tired.

(*Neither* LIZZIE *nor* NELLIE *goes.*)

CELINE   Can I have that iron when you're done with it, Vera?

VERA   O.K.

THELMA   [*to* CELINE] Boy, did I get yelled at this morning!

CELINE   You! They even yell at me when I follow the rules. I think they like you better when you break them.

THELMA   Yeah, but I don't even know the rules yet.

(THELMA *is a new arrival on the ward.*)

JULIA   Say, Celine, when are you going to stop being a ward warmer and go to work?

CELINE   You should talk, I don't see you doing anything.

JULIA   I got my things to do, but all you do is get on everyone else's nerves.

CELINE   You can slam me all you want, Julia. I'm waiting to go to work on Companion Service. You're just after me because I don't work and because Mrs. Talbot said I didn't have to.

(JULIA *does not reply but turns to talk with* BETTY, *the patient in charge of cleaning the ward.*)

CELINE   At least I take a bath and don't leave my clothes hanging up in the bathroom.

JULIA   The other girls work and can't take a bath until the night. That's their excuse.

(JULIA *leaves.*)

ELIZABETH   [*speaking to no one in particular*] I don't think she [JULIA] likes me, although she trades cigarettes for coffee with me. She never did like me. We were together on Ward 4.

11:00 A.M. Medication time. Mrs. Bender sticks her head out of the nurses' office: "O.K., ladies, it's medicine time." Julia is walking by the office.

MRS. BENDER   Julia, will you call the girls in the loggia for their medicine?

JULIA   What for? I don't work here, that's your job.

MRS. BENDER   Well, thanks a lot.

JULIA   You're quite welcome.

(CELINE *appears on the scene and goes out to the loggia to call the other patients.*)

12:15 P.M. Dinnertime. The patients leave in a group with the patients from Ward Y upstairs. They are alternately accompanied by a Ward X attendant or a Ward Y attendant. After dinner the patients return separately. Some return to work, others off to a variety of places—beauty shop (every other Thursday), bowling or skating in town (about once a month), canteen, recreation center, typing classes, art classes, laundry ("you can take your good things to special people at the laundry and pay them for it. They don't throw your stuff in with everything else."), social worker, or chaplain are some of the places patients generally spend free time during the day.

4:00 P.M. Roll call. The evening shift attendant, Mrs. Minton, comes on duty. There is a transfer of keys and important information between shifts. After roll call the patients are usually on the ward until suppertime. All patients are back on the ward, except dining room workers who work the evening meal.

5:15 P.M. Supper hour. Once again all patients leave in a group, but this time they return in a group. Mrs. Minton, the evening attendant, feels that this is the only way to get all patients back for medication.

5:45 P.M. Medication. Following this, patients bathe and dress for evening activities. All activities are attended in a group and returned from in a group. Available activities include dances, social hour of cards, ping-pong, shuffleboard, ball games in the summer, and movies on Friday and Saturday evening.

All patients not attending activities must remain on the ward, where they watch television, read, write letters, do their laundry, or go to bed. Very few patients remain on the ward when activities are available.

9:00 P.M. Patients return from activities. They either watch television, prepare for bed, or sit in the loggia smoking and talking.

MAUREEN   How was the dance tonight, Julia?

JULIA   Didn't you go? What happened?

MAUREEN   I decided to stay in and wash some things out.

JULIA   I was going to wash my hair tonight.

MAUREEN   I'm going to my sister's for the weekend.

JULIA   Is Doctor Powell really letting you go? I'll believe that when I see it.

JULIA   Gee, it's quiet in here. How come you don't play the piano any more, Elizabeth?

ELIZABETH   I don't know. At night all I think about is washing my face, and during the day all I think about is mail.

JULIA   Four hours to wash your face! Why don't you wash it and get it over with?

ELIZABETH   That's a pretty dress you have on tonight, Clara.

RUTH   Do I owe you any cigarettes, Elizabeth?

ELIZABETH   No. No one owes me coffee or cigarettes.

RUTH   Well, can I borrow one then 'till tomorrow? I'll pay you back.

(JULIA *goes into the dayroom. She leaves her cigarette in the ashtray. While she is gone,* MARILYN, *a very disturbed patient, comes into the loggia. She sits in* JULIA'S *chair and starts smoking* JULIA'S *cigarette.* JULIA *returns.*)

JULIA   Did you pick up that goddamn cigarette?

BETTY   Well, she don't know any better, the way she is. Besides, there was no name on it.

JULIA   Goddamn son-of-a-bitch, there was Pall Mall on it.

(*Patients on the loggia break into laughter.* JULIA *leaves.*)

LELA   That Julia. I just love to hear her talk. She is something. And dance, you should see her. She doesn't go to the dances often, but when she does, she really dances.

10:00 P.M. Bedtime and lights out. Mrs. Minton straightens out the ward, sweeps, picks up papers, and empties ashtrays.

11:45 P.M. Mrs. Calen, the night shift attendant, comes on duty.

Patient Adaptations

The patient world can be considered a world of "unfreedom." Almost every detail of life for the patient is subject to the scrutiny, comment, or control of others. Patients are told when to rise, when to sleep, what to wear, what to eat, how to talk, how to act, who to talk to, and even how to think. They are dependent upon the hospital for their food, clothing, cigarettes, and toiletries. Material possessions and goods that are taken for granted at almost every level of living outside the institution are transformed into scarce commodities. In most of these respects, the mental hospital closely resembles the prison. Both institutions have been characterized by Goffman as "total institutions," a concept that reflects our description of the world of unfreedom.[2]

There is, however, an additional element in our use of "unfreedom." In the mental hospital, as well as the prison, there is a conscious attempt at destruction of the patient's self that existed prior to institutionalization.[3] The self that existed prior to hospitalization is defined as having been in some way the cause of the patient's present condition. Thus, the old self must be destroyed, and a new self incorporated through a resocialization process. This process begins with a stage of "status homogenization" in which patients are reduced to a condition of forced equality that tolerates no expression of purely individual needs.

In this section, we will characterize the system of social relationships on the ward—its norms, attitudes, and beliefs—as a response to the condition of unfreedom. We assume the existence of strains created by this loss of freedom, and view the emergence of certain normative patterns as a response.

THE NATURE OF PATIENT NORMS

Normative prescriptions for behavior are generally viewed as having some moral foundation. One is enjoined to behave in certain ways because it is "just" or "right." Internal compulsions or external pressures ensure the group definitions of desirable behavior. In many ways, some of the normative patterns that will be described do not contain any overall shared group definition of "right" behavior. Thus, for certain norms there is no definite constraint to

---

[2] See Erving Goffman, *Asylums* (New York: Doubleday-Anchor, 1961).

[3] Goffman also treats this point under the more general process of "self-mortification."

behave in a specified way. We have viewed the emergence of various
behavior patterns as a response to the strains of living in a state of
unfreedom. Once these patterns are selected by a patient, they then
become his social self. He is reacted to by both patients and staff
according to his initial behavior and is from that time on under a
group definition of appropriate behavior.

The relative absence of shared group definitions regarding normative behavior reveals a significant feature of the patient world. It
can best be seen by contrasting inmate norms in a prison. In prison
life, the very foundation underlying the development of inmate
norms is the existence of a clearly defined outgroup or enemy,
namely the staff.[4] The antagonisms that exist between inmates and
staff is the core about which other normative patterns develop. Although deviations from other inmate norms may be tolerated, norms
proscribing cooperation with prison staff are strictly enforced. The
development of a peculiar inmate language—its argot and jargon—
is added evidence of the gap that exists between inmate and staff.

The existence of a peculiar language form used by patients is
conspicuous by its absence on Ward X. If anything, there is more of
an attempt to use the language of the staff in characterizing or discussing fellow patients. The absence of these patterns is consistent
with the fact that the staff on Ward X is not defined as the enemy.
Group cohesion among the patients does not have this source of
support, as is found in the prison. Patients generally accept the
definition that the staff are there to help them. When an attendant
tells a patient to do something, she is doing it for the patient's own
good. This positive orientation toward the staff, however, is not
without a strong covert suspicion of staff motives—a suspicion which,
though not openly expressed by the majority of patients, is nevertheless present in many patient conversations. For example, Wanda, in
commenting on how several patients are always talking against Dr.
Powell: "I don't like to listen to them when they talk like that; it
upsets me. I don't know what I'd do if I didn't believe that Dr.
Powell was really trying to help me." Nora, in defending the motives
of attendants: "I think most of the attendants here are really concerned about us patients. Some people here say that the attendants
are only here for their eight hours and their money, but I don't

[4] See, e.g., Donald Clemmer, *The Prison Community* (Boston: Christo-
pher Publishing House, 1940).

agree." Maureen: "The attendants are really interested in caring for you while you are here, but I don't think they're that interested in my general welfare. [Observer: What do you mean by your general welfare?] Well, you know, in my being somebody, or having something."

These examples reflect the general nature of many patients' responses when they are asked to interpret the motives of staff personnel. In spite of the favorable nature of the response, there is generally introduced some question regarding staff motives which most patients impute to other patients. The covert form of this suspicion also seems clear. For if a patient openly rejects the idea that the staff is working for the good of the patient, then he must also accept the hopelessness of his situation. In most cases, this is too threatening to accept. At the same time, however, it is difficult to view the staff as totally altruistic and benevolent when they are responsible for the very conditions of unfreedom that sometimes makes hospital life difficult for the patients. The ambivalence in this situation is likely to produce more latent anxiety and aggression than would be found in a situation in which the "enemy" is clearly defined.[5] In many ways, the ambivalence is difficult for the patient to handle, and may provide support of existing pathological thought processes of certain patients (see, e.g., Cameron's discussion of the "paranoid pseudocommunity").[6]

THE NORMS THEMSELVES

The classification of patient norms must be made along some dimension. Alternatives for classification may include the distribution of the norms, the strength of the sanctions attached to the norms, or the transmission of norms.[7] We shall classify patient

[5] Cloward has pointed to the role of the inmate system as a means of avoiding the internalization of outgroup definitions. See Richard A. Cloward, "Social Control in the Prison," in *Theoretical Studies in Social Organization of the Prison*, Social Science Research Council, Pamphlet 15 (March 1960), p. 21.

[6] Norman Cameron, "The Paranoid Pseudo-Community," *American Journal of Sociology*, Vol. 49 (July 1943), 32–38.

[7] See, e.g., Richard T. Morris, "A Typology of Norms," *American Sociological Review*, 21 (October 1956), 610–13.

norms along a content dimension, namely, the nature of the action called for by the norms as well as the area of behavior that is being regulated. Broadly speaking, the former refers to whether the norm directs patients to participate in a certain way or whether to avoid certain behavior. The latter refers to whether the norm focuses upon the self or upon self-other relationships. Let us now turn to the norms themselves.

NORMS OF ACCOMMODATION

Norms of accommodation refer to the acceptance of formal ward rules as they are set forth by the ward staff. The activation of these norms by patients allows them to make their peace with the institution because they assure the staff of maximum predictability for ward routine. "The best way to get along around here is to co-operate with the attendants whether you agree with their ideas or not," said one patient. Another remarked, "The first thing a new girl has to learn around here is to do what they tell you." "Doing what they tell you" generally refers to: "never go off the ward without signing out; make sure you walk to eat with the ward; they don't like it if you don't keep your room clean around here; you have to make sure you know when and where to smoke; everyone should do some work here in the hospital—it helps out the attendants and it keeps your mind off your own troubles."

Patients are aware, however, that compliance with accommodation norms can also yield extra privileges of various sorts. For example, a cooperative patient may get coffee from the attendants, or permission to lie down in his room during the day, or permission to go to activities off grounds. The more perceptive patient is able to see the rewards that go beyond the distribution of extra privileges: "If you can get close enough to an attendant, then maybe you can make her understand how you are when you get upset. That way, you can get to talk to the attendant when you are upset," or "[If you're a good patient] when you get into an argument with another patient, the attendant will usually take your part."

Thus, accommodative norms are not necessarily exhibited by patients because they are valued in and of themselves. Compliance with such norms can result in extra privileges. On the other hand, compliance by patients with norms prescribing hospital work that is highly valued by staff is also valued by the patients. For the staff, working patients are essential for the operation of the hospital. For the patients, the work role allows them to occasionally drop the patient role as well as to provide them with a release from the boredom of ward life.

NORMS OF DISSOCIATION

"One of the first things a new girl learns around here is to stay away from the other patients. Don't ask them questions or ask for advice. Take that Celine. She's a bureau of misinformation. Always talking about what she knows about the hospital, and she's usually wrong." This comment by a Ward X patient reflects the nature of certain types of patient norms which function to discourage the emergence of stable relationships among patients. The norms referred to generally discourage belief in the information heard from patients, with the idea that if you seek to act in terms of this information, the result can only be trouble for the patient. Thus, though many patients engage in exchange of hearsay and gossip, there is much bickering over the credibility of the information.

The consequence of such norms, which discourage a belief in the content of the information exchanged among patients, is a sort of voluntary isolation. As one patient put it: "It's real hard to know what's going on here, because you can't ask too many questions. If you ask the other girls, they don't give you accurate answers. If you ask the attendants too many questions, they get upset with so many patients to handle. The best way is to keep to yourself and just feel your way around." This type of isolation is also encouraged by staff in telling patients to "worry about yourself, and stop getting all wrapped up in someone else's troubles."

Aside from these norms which directly discourage involvement among patients, there is another normative pattern which has the same latent function. These are what we might generally call norms of privacy. Herein we find strong taboos against talking about your own illness or another patient's illness. This taboo extends to even the most disturbed patients, in that the behavior of patients who are "climbing the walls" is tolerated but not discussed. When a disturbed patient violates the property or person of another patient, she is protected by an awareness that "she doesn't know what she's doing."

Along with taboos against discussing patients' conditions, there is also a strong reluctance to talk of one's past or life outside the hospital. Patients do not discuss their families or the families of others. In many ways, these privacy norms would seem to be reactions to the lack of privacy that patients have in their relations to staff. Patients are, so to speak, "laid bare" by the staff; their illness, family, and anything else known concerning the patient are the routine subject matter for staff in their work with patients.[8] Thus, the privacy norms among patients are apparent attempts to avoid complete exposure to fellow patients.

NORMS OF STATUS MAINTENANCE

In our earlier discussion of the condition of unfreedom as it exists on Ward X, we spoke of the process of destruction of the self and the loss of one's larger society status. Cloward, in discussing the prison, has spoken of the process of "status degradation" that confronts the prison inmate.[9] The norms we shall now speak of relate to attempts of patients to maintain a favorable self-image or sense of personal worth.

It is perhaps unfortunate that many patient attempts at status maintenance are often interpreted by staff as nothing more than uncooperativeness, belligerence, or a pathological disturbance. However, even the most cooperative and docile patient may make an

---

[8] Other examples of this lack of privacy may even be found in the interview situations between the ward physician and a patient. When a patient requests to see the doctor during his daily ward visit the interview takes place in the nurses' office. During the interview either one or both of the attendants are present, as well as the ward nurse. Similarly, during "ward rounds" (when the doctor goes from patient to patient in the dayroom to answer questions), the questions and requests of patients are made in the presence of all the other patients as well as the staff.

[9] In this connection see Cloward, "Social Control in the Prison"; and Harold Garfinkle, "Conditions of Successful Degradation Ceremonies," *American Journal of Sociology*, 61 (March 1956), 420–24.

attempt at status maintenance. The following situations illustrate what we mean by status-maintenance norms.

(Nora has been called in to see Dr. Powell. She has been reported to have been keeping company with a male patient who has been the alleged cause of several patient pregnancies.)

DR. POWELL   I guess if you want to take the position that you'll show the hospital what you can and can't do, that's your business. But you can't expect them not to talk.

NORA   Well, it's none of that attendant's business. She's all the time trying to mother me.

DR. POWELL   Well, kid, if you want to do it, I guess it's your business.

NORA   Don't call me kid. People have gotten in trouble with me for less.

DR. POWELL   Well, I can't call you Mrs., because you're not married. How about Ma'am?

NORA   No! I'm no school marm.

DR. POWELL   What shall I call you then? Miss?

NORA   You could try calling me Nora.

Here we see what appears to be an attempt on the part of the patient to be responded to as a person separate from her patient role. We can see a similar response in the following illustrations.

(During ward round, Dr. Powell goes from patient to patient in the dayroom inquiring about the present state of their health, or answering questions on matters of concern to a patient.)

DR. POWELL   Well, here's Julia. How are you functioning today, Julia?

JULIA   Functioning! What the hell do you think I am, a machine? I don't function, I breathe and think. You can't understand that, can you?

The other aspect of attempts at status maintenance is found in patients' reluctance to discard the way of life they knew prior to hospitalization. This usually results in internal tensions and conflicts, because, as we suggested earlier, the staff generally defines a patient's prehospital life as "causing" the present pathological state. For example, one patient commented:

They always resented me here because I was different from everyone else. I have different interests like athletics, sewing, dancing and reading. The same thing happens when 1 talk about how I used to live. I can't help it. I like to remember my earlier life. They were good years. They always throw it up to me about the things I had before I came to this place. Once the social workers said to me, "Isn't it a shame that you'll never have rugs on your floor again?" It's the same with the doctor, he's always saying that I should forget my past glories.

It should be noted that our purpose here is not to question the therapeutic purpose or effectiveness of staff policy regarding a patient's way of life prior to hospitalization. We only wish to demonstrate patients' reactions to such a policy, and the way the policy may become infused with values pertaining to maintaining status distinctions between staff and patients. The latter point is revealed in the following incident:

(*After morning roll call, one of the patients goes directly to the signout desk and begins to enter her name in the book. The attendant walks over to her.*)

ATTENDANT   You're in a big hurry this morning. Where are you going?
PATIENT   I've got a date to play tennis with Fred. [PATIENT *uses the first name of staff member in recreation department.*]
ATTENDANT   Well, in the first place, his name is Mr. Borton. And in the second place, we need help on the ward. If you're well enough to play tennis, you're well enough to help clean the ward.

These, then, are examples of behavior which reflect norms of status maintenance, and of staff reactions to such behavior. Basically, these norms are departures from the formal patient role and from the traditional low status of patients in the hierarchy.

NORMS OF IMPROVEMENT

Under the heading of norms of improvement, what we find is a recognition, on the part of the patient, of one's illness and a definite desire to accept the help of staff personnel in working toward recovery. Patients who state, "I know I'm not well and I'm going to do everything the doctor tells me to do so I can get better," illustrate the activation of this norm. These patients, in effect, put themselves completely in the hands of the staff.

Few patients, however, actively orient themselves around norms of improvement. For one thing, most patients on Ward X have been in the hospital for more than five years. This factor tends to make it difficult for a patient to persist in his adherence to improvement norms. Second, there are many patients who would gladly accept staff help for improvement but who would not entirely accept their illness. For example, one patient who had just agreed to see the ward doctor once a week for individual therapy stated: "Let's not call it therapy, doctor, let's just say we are talking together."

These factors, plus the relative absence of a vigorous treatment milieu and the understaffing problem, provides very little foundation for the maintenance and persistence of norms of improvement.

What we have suggested in this section regarding patient norms is (1) that certain strains resulting from the state of unfreedom give rise to different normative patterns which function to mitigate strains; (2) that the patterns discussed are not norms in the sense that all patients are under pressure to activate *all* norms, but rather that they represent alternative modes of adaptation to the situation; and (3) that once a mode of adaptation is selected and activated, a patient creates his "niche" (i.e., role) on the ward, and is from that time on under group pressure to exhibit behavior consistent with his selection.

MODES OF ADAPTATION

Implicit in the nature of the norms described above are several possible modes of adaptation available to the patients on Ward X. An adaptation may be viewed as the way in which a patient "chooses" to "fit into" the hospital world. We shall not be concerned with the conditions which give rise to one or another adaptation; but simply to describe four ideal-typical adjustments that patients make to their social environment. The four adaptations are withdrawal, accommodation, conversion, and resistance.

The *withdrawal* mode of adaptation is essentially a flight from the situation. Patients in this category are for the most part entirely asocial. They neither initiate interaction nor do they respond to interaction directed to them. They are not necessarily psychologically withdrawn, however, for many of the patients falling into this category are quite intact.[10] Their withdrawal is seen in the absence of relationships of any sort with those about them. It should also be noted that while these patients isolate themselves from both other patients and staff, they are still quite cooperative with respect to hospital and ward rules. However, it might even be misleading to call their behavior cooperative, because they perform all the expected behaviors without ever really being asked. You can always be sure that their beds will be made, that they will be present for roll call and for medications, that they will keep their rooms clean, and so forth. Their compliance in these areas, however, is not given with the expectation of receiving "something extra" for their cooperation. They are quite removed from susceptibility to any such motivational structure.

The *accommodation* mode of adaptation is found with the patients who conform to the expectations of both the staff and the other patients. Here we find the staff definition of the "perfect patient" or the patient definition of a "good gal." With accommodation we find a moderately active patient. Very little interaction is initiated by these patients, but they are excellent targets for interactions—they are "good listeners." Accommodation also implies that these patients neither question, defend, nor attack things said to them by either patients or staff. In the absence of any definite response to the behavior directed toward them these patients tend to be quite supportive in their relations with others. In effect, the absence of response can be freely interpreted as agreement.

Thus, patients operating under this mode have a relatively harmonious existence on the ward, an existence which has been earned at the expense of never making a demand, voicing an opinion, or making a negative or positive comment about others. For example, the responses to the following questions most closely resemble this ideal-typical mode of adaptation.

[10] One striking example is the case of a patient who was a social isolate and rarely spoke to anyone on the ward. Early in the study she was identified to the observer as one of the "withdrawn" patients. During a psychodrama session conducted by a visiting psychologist, this patient was purposely selected for "role playing" in order to see if the psychodrama had any impact on her. Much to the surprise of ward staff, she gave a rather verbal and imaginative performance with only a minimum of prompting.

Q. How do you think the ward physician would like you to act most of the time?

A. Oh, I don't know. I try to do what the other girls do.

Q. What differences are there between the attendants on the three shifts?

A. Well, they're all pretty busy, but they're about the same.

Q. When a patient on this ward does something that really bothers you, what do you do about it?

A. Get up and leave them.

Q. There are many fine nurses here in the hospital. If you had a choice, who would you choose as the best nurse?

A. I have never talked with many nurses, so I don't know.

We find in these responses a noncommittal orientation to events on the ward. Obviously, there are departures from this pattern, but when measured relative to the responses of other patients, they are, on the whole, more of an accommodation mode of adaptation than any other. For purposes of clarity, let us look at the responses to the first question given by patients operating under other modes of adaptation.

Q. How do you think the ward physician would like you to act most of the time?

Conversion:

A. He expects you to obey and to do what he tells you. Mind the attendants and the supervisor. If you don't, he'll have to pull you off the ward.

Resistance:

A. I really don't know. One time he says one thing and the next time another. Whenever there's a crowd around, he starts that same old stuff, "Oh, everybody here knows Mrs. _____!" Then he goes and tells everything about me. That's one thing I can't stand about him.

With the *conversion* mode of adaptation we find patients who indicate a strong identification with the staff. Much of their behavior on the ward is imitative of staff behavior. For example, the conversion response to the question indicated above is an attendant's standard rationale for persuading patients to obey certain orders.

Patients operating under this mode of adaptation literally "bend over backwards" to help ward staff members. They will convey information, run errands, do ward chores, and in general, "hang around ward personnel all day." With the conversion mode of adaptation there is also a relatively marked amount of contact between patients and staff. With this contact, patients operating under this mode have greater access to the values, attitudes, and beliefs of the staff. Given this information, these patients generally espouse and support staff norms much more religiously than do the staff members themselves.

There is, however, a curious relationship between ward staff and conversion patients. On the one hand, staff is quite appreciative of their help, but on the other hand, they resent the status advances made by these patients. The following statement by a ward attendant reflects this ambivalence.

Dr. Powell and Dr. Hand told me to keep an eye on Lynn M.'s menstrual cycle because it was very erratic. I figured Betty L. would be good to do this, because she can really handle some of these girls. Well, what do you think Betty did, she sent a note directly to Dr. Hand about Lynn's condition. I've got to make her understand that she can't go over my head whenever she feels like it. That's her trouble. She's too pushy. She would take over this ward if you'd let her.

This is the problem faced by the ward attendants, who, while becoming dependent upon conversion patients, must also maintain the traditional staff-patient separateness. Many patients, on the other hand, are openly hostile toward the conversion patients. They resent being ordered around by, watched by, or responsible to other patients who have no ties to the patient world.

The last mode of adaptation is *resistance*. Here we find behavior ranging from a calm and serious questioning of the shortcomings of hospital procedures and facilities to an outright rejection of the authority, motives, and competence of ward staff personnel. Patients operating under this mode are greatly concerned with maintaining their own self-respect and dignity. In this respect, they resist all efforts to place them in the general category of patient.

This does not mean that resistance patients do not comply with formal ward rules. They still take their medication, sign out for roll call, and clean their rooms. The differences are that (1) they view these necessary activities as artificially imposed rules that can be and should be changed, and (2) they will not accept staff authority to "spread" into areas they consider beyond the necessary limits of staff control, such as telling a patient how to dress and use makeup, or indicating which patients to be friendly with, or what kinds of books they should or should not read.

A concern with status maintenance leads many resistance patients to avoid anything that may result in close ties with staff. One patient, for example, remarked: "The staff will try to win you over here; and if they're successful it usually works against you. If you get too chummy with the doctor, the other patients call you a pet and they lose respect for you. If you get too chummy with the attendants, they will load their work on you."

Concern with the respect of other patients is also important, for resistance patients receive considerable covert and subtle support from other patients. Thus, they enjoy a very high position within the patient group. This fact is quite curious, however, in that resistance patients do not really consider themselves a part of the patient group; their identifications are not wholly confined to other patients, and they may quite openly reject many patient norms. We shall return to this particular point in the next chapter.

In this chapter we have tried to describe the main outlines of hospital routine, the dominant patient norms found on Ward X, and four modes of adaptation to hospital life exhibited by patients. It seems clear from this material that whatever the value of hospitalization, it does not provide patients with freedom from the stress and strain of daily life so as to enable them to devote all their time and energies to treatment and rehabilitation. Patients continue to experience the demands of occupational roles, pseudo-familial roles, economic scarcity, political powerlessness, and interpersonal adjustments. If difficulty in facing the demands of living with limited choices and resources is part of the reason why people are in mental hospitals, they unfortunately must face the same situation when they get there.

4

The Hospital Caste System

The internal social structure of the mental hospital is a product of several factors, each of which was identified earlier. First is the caste-like structure of the hospital which sets up formidable barriers to close interpersonal relationships between persons in different positions in the hierarchy. Second is the vulnerability of persons in authority to challenges to their authority because of their inability to demonstrate and use their expertise to gain respect and compliance from others. Third is the absence of clear, attainable goals for patients and staff regarding treatment, cure, and release. And finally, there is the inevitable and indispensable daily interaction that takes place among patients and staff in the hospital that represent departures from formal organizational roles. Taken together, these elements put considerable pressure on the formal structure of the hospital and serve to produce the unique features of daily hospital life.

In the preceding chapter we described some of the factors that work against the emergence of a strong inmate culture that has its own binding codes, norms, and special vocabulary. Norms of dissociation, norms of privacy, and ambivalent attitudes of patients toward staff were cited as factors which operate to maintain a "separateness" among patients. Similarly, the modes of accommodation exhibited by patients reflect either a withdrawal from other patients or an orientation toward staff. Regardless of the particular adaptation selected, it is an individual and not a collective adaptation. In addition to the absence of a distinctive patient subculture, there is no stable status structure that is based upon adherence to patient-supported norms.

There is, however, a strong tendency toward organization among patients that is a by-product of the staff's pursuit of day-to-day custodial goals and the rigid caste structure which influences social relationships. Attendants, for example, must be concerned with the custodial goals of the institution. In order for the ward and hospital to operate effectively, patients must be motivated to work, to keep their rooms clean, to take medication, to sign in and sign out, and, in general, to comply with numerous ward rules. In the process of motivating patients, attendants distribute rewards and privileges for varying degrees of cooperation. Certain patients are allowed to control and "ride herd" over other patients in return for more effective control of patients. Scarce goods are given to patients in return for information about which particular patients are not taking their medication or who has been going behind the MS Building with male patients. In the process of exchange of rewards for cooperation and exceptional behavior (i.e., behavior that patients are not formally required to exhibit), a basis for repeated violation of caste lines is established.

What we are suggesting, then, is that among patients a status hierarchy along a dimension of patient norms does not exist. On the contrary, patients are located in a hierarchy, and are differentially responded to along a dimension of *contact* with *staff* groups. A patient's position in the status structure is viewed as a function of (1) her access to prestigious groups—i.e., staff, along a purely quantitative dimension; (2) her access to prestigious symbols of upper-level staff groups—i.e., knowledge of private and public information concerning staff members; and (3) the qualitative nature of her contacts with staff.

These three elements defining a patient's position within the patient status hierarchy may be combined under the general heading of social distance patterns. Several recent studies of formal organizations or of formal authority relationships have given a central position to the concept of social distance. Seeman and Evans,[1]

[1] Melvin Seeman and John W. Evans, "Stratification and Hospital Care: I. The Performance of the Medical Interne," *American Sociological Review*, 26 (February 1961), 67–80.

Pearlin and Rosenberg,[2] Kadushin,[3] and Segal [4] have all investigated the organizational consequences of various patterns of social distance in interstatus relationships. What has been notably lacking, as Seeman and Evans point out, is an attempt to formulate a theory of intraorganization stratification. In this chapter we explore the outlines of such a theory by examining the social distance strategies employed in interstatus relationships on a psychiatric ward.

We are treating the patient social structure as exemplary of our general view of intraorganization stratification systems. For example, the organization may be seen as a network of social distance patterns about a set of fixed positions. Moreover, the distance patterns may be seen as interconnected, such that the "closeness" or "distance" in a relationship (say, between B and C, where B is a higher position than C) is directly related to the closeness or distance in the relation between person B and his superordinate. More concretely, the greater the social distance between a doctor and an attendant, the greater the social distance between the attendant and the patients. We assume that each person in the organization is concerned with maintaining or advancing his position within the structure.[5] The set of actions following from these assumptions

[2] Leonard I. Pearlin and Morris Rosenberg, "Nurse-Patient Social Distance and the Structural Context of a Mental Hospital," *American Sociological Review*, 27 (February 1962), 56–65.

[3] Charles Kadushin, "Social Distance Between Client and Professional," *American Journal of Sociology*, 67 (March 1962), 517–31.

[4] Bernard E. Segal, "Nurses and Patients: Time, Place, and Distance," *Social Problems*, 9 (Winter 1962), 257–64.

[5] The formal structure of hospitals is characterized by what Harvey L. Smith has called "blocked mobility." ("The Sociological Study of Hospitals," unpublished Ph.D. dissertation, University of Chicago, 1949.) The distinction between an organization that "feeds on itself" (i.e., provides for internal mobility) and an organization characterized by blocked mobility has a number of important implications for the authority structure of the organization. For example, in the first organization provisions have to be made for diffusing knowledge and information (e.g., informal norms) for the purpose of making job changes in the organization without necessarily impairing its operating effectiveness. Where mobility is blocked, as in the psychiatric hospital, we would expect to find substitutes for promotion in the form of seeking significant social contacts and reducing social distance from superordinates.

are (1) maximizing social distance with respect to subordinates and minimizing social distance with respect to superordinates; (2) maintaining a clear distinction between public and private symbols— i.e., formal organizational self and extraorganizational self; and (3) distributing rewards (i.e., contacts with subordinates) in a way that contributes to the maintenance of social distance.[6]

In this chapter we shall use this framework to examine the interrelated nature of the social distance patterns among patients and staff. The following section contains a look at the status structure among the study ward patients as revealed by positive and negative sociometric choices. A patient's position within the patient group will then be analyzed in terms of the nature of contact with higher status groups.[7]

[6] The utility of this framework was explored in an examination of interlocking social distance patterns on all psychiatric wards at Riverview Hospital. It was found that attendants who perceived greater social distance from their superordinates (i.e., doctors and nurses) were more likely to maximize social distance from their subordinates (i.e., patients). This relationship was found in different structural contexts of the hospital (open and closed wards, day and night shifts) where the social accessibility of superordinates was limited, and where the status aggression of the subordinates was the greatest. Different social distance strategies on the part of attendants were seen either as attempts to enhance status or as protective mechanisms against positional threats.

[7] The study ward is composed of patients who are considered to be "somewhere between the hospital and the community," and are viewed as having "manageable symptoms." Selected aspects of the ward and the patient population were described in Chapter Three.

Sociometric Choices and Group Structure

A sociometric questionnaire was used to determine the main outlines of the status system on Ward X.[8] Patients were asked to

[8] The observer asked each of the patients on the ward if they would talk with him. He stressed the voluntary nature of their cooperation. Of the 54 patients on the ward, 29 agreed to fill out a sociometric questionnaire. Almost all of the 25 patients who refused to participate were those who were generally inaccessible to ward personnel. They spent most of their time in their rooms or in isolated-sedentary activities. Compared to the participating patients, the nonparticipants were on the average older (43 to 53 years), and their present illness was of longer duration (7 years to 10 years). There were no differences by education or formal diagnosis.

select two persons who would be very desirable roommates, two who would be undesirable roommates, and one person for a position of leadership on the ward.[9] Almost all the persons named on the questionnaires were from among those patients who agreed to cooperate with the observer by completing the questionnaire.[10]

In the distribution of positive roommate choices, we found a rather wide dispersion of choices; 22 of the 29 patients received at least one choice. Fifty percent of the choices were distributed among 7 patients, and we found 9 mutually choosing pairs, 1 perfect triad, and 1 near-perfect triad.

In contrast, the distribution of negative roommate choices indicated a marked pattern of convergence. Fifteen of the 29 patients received at least one negative choice, with over 50 percent of the choices falling to 4 patients. An even more marked pattern of concentration characterized the distribution of leadership choices. Only 11 of the 29 patients received at least one leadership choice, and 50 percent of the choices were concentrated on 2 patients.

Thus, we have isolated those patients who are high on positive roommate choices, high on negative roommate choices, and high on leadership choices. The question we now raise is: Can quantity and quality of staff-patient contacts explain the relative positions of these patients? In line with our earlier comments, the nature of the contacts will be discussed in terms of their consequences for maintaining social distance patterns within and between patient-staff status groups.

Table 4-1 shows the distribution of the quantity and quality of contacts with staff for each patient within the three sociometric groups. Quantity of contacts, or "contact ratio," is the ratio of the total number of contacts to the number of hours for which

[9] The questions respectively were: "If you were given a choice of the two girls on your ward you would most like to room with, which two girls would you choose?"; "Which two girls on your ward would you least like to room with?"; "If you were on a committee in charge of a party on your ward, which girl from your ward would you choose to be chairman of the committee?"

[10] Because the sociometric questionnaire was not administered in a group setting, the low number of choices received by patients who did not participate in filling out the questionnaire was probably not a result of their failure to participate.

TABLE 4-1

THE AMOUNT AND CONTENT OF STAFF-PATIENT CONTACT BY SELECTED SOCIOMETRIC CHOICES

Group	Contact Ratio	Total Number of Contacts[a]	Content of Contact				
			Attention and Information	Service Request	Staff Favors	Criticism	Formal Business
Hi Positives:[b]	$\bar{X}$ = .29						
Elizabeth K.	.28	16	10	3	1	2	..
Mary G.	.20	10	8	2	..	..	..
Cathy D.	.00	0	..	..	..	..	..
Joan B.	.61	34	19	9	1	3	2
Annie G.	.18	9	5	3	1	..	..
Wanda R.	.46	27	16	6	5	..	..
Hi Negatives:[c]	$\bar{X}$ = 1.04						
Celine B.	1.28	72	43	9	20	..	..
Betty L.	1.25	70	40	10	12	2	6
Ruth C.	.28	17	11	..	4	2	..
Lizzie S.	1.35	70	38	12	20	..	..
Hi Leaders:[d]	$\bar{X}$ = 1.61						
Nora P.	1.04	63	18	4	5	6	30
Julia T.	2.18	122	68	17	3	23	11

a Absolute number of contacts.
b Whom would you most like to room with?
c Whom would you least like to room with?
d Whom would you choose to be chairman of a committee?

contact interaction was recorded (56 hours). Contacts were classified according to the nature of the contact situation.[11]

Inspection of Table 4-1 reveals rather marked similarities of contact pattern *within* each sociometric group. With few exceptions, persons in each group tend to exhibit similar overall contact ratios. In addition, the content of the contact *within* each

[11] Examples of each qualitative category are as follows (in each case the contact is from the patient to the staff members):

Attention and Information

"Do I have a canteen card this week?"
"Can I get on the beauty shop list?"

Service Requests

"Will you shave my legs, Mrs. Bender?"
"Will someone open my room for me?"

Staff Favors

"Can I get your lunch today?"
"I'll go over and pick up the medicine basket."

Criticism

"No, I don't want any cigarette paper. I don't smoke that crap the state hands out."
"You can't even burp around here without it being written down."

(Refers to the fact that soda mints given to patients must be charted.)

Formal Business

"Would you see to it that this notice is read at evening roll call?"
"The next inter-ward council meeting will be held here, so we'll have to prepare for it."

After the author coded the content of the contact into one of the above categories, 20 contacts were randomly selected from each category and submitted to another judge for classification. There was agreement on 78 of the 100 contacts. The distribution of the 22 errors did not indicate a concentration in certain categories.

group tends to be located in the same categories. This supports our assumption concerning the contact-with-staff basis for the patient status hierarchy.

"Hi Positives," who have a relatively low average contact ratio, tend to concentrate their contacts in the rather formalized areas of "Attention and Information" and "Service Requests." Contacts in each of these areas can be viewed as being within formal organizational bounds: the interaction situation is such that participants may maintain and reinforce the distinctions inherent in the formal patient-staff positions. Contacts in the other three content areas, which involve departures from formal roles on the part of either or both staff and patients, are almost nonexistent.

"Hi Negatives," who have relatively high average contact ratio, show a considerable number of contacts in the area of "Staff Favors." This is in marked contrast to the almost total absence of "Staff Favors" contacts in the other two sociometric groups.

Turning to the "Hi Leaders" we see a shift to the areas of "Criticism" and "Formal Business." They also have the highest contact ratios in all areas except "Staff Favors."

These different patterns of staff contact in each of the three status groups can be translated, we believe, into three distinct social distance patterns between staff and patients. Each social distance pattern, in turn, poses a different problem for the staff, who are on the receiving end of the contacts and distance patterns, and for the patients from whom the contacts emanate. For example, we shall try to show that "Hi Positives" do not pose a threat to the ward staff or the patients. "Hi Negatives," on the other hand, pose a *status threat* to both staff and patients. "Hi Leaders" are viewed as posing a *power threat* to the staff and providing status enhancement for patients.

If the presence of such threats is real for the staff, then we would expect to find that certain staff reactions seek to minimize the threat. Such reactions will be examined in terms of staff attempts to maximize social distance between themselves and the patients.

STATUS THREATS, POWER THREATS, AND SOCIAL DISTANCE

In this section we shall speak of status threats and power threats as two types of strategy patients employ to close the "gap" between themselves and ward staff. (It should be kept in mind that these features are part of our general concern with the internal structure of a mental hospital. In the next chapter, the same processes will be shown to operate in staff-staff relationships.) Status threats involve attempts to gain knowledge of staff's extraorganizational self, or access to *private symbols*—e.g., first-name interaction, discussions of families and home life, and personal discussions of attitudes toward the hospital in general and other staff in particular.

Power threats, on the other hand, involve attempts to gain knowledge primarily of the staff's organizational self, or access to *public symbols*—e.g., knowledge of formal rules, knowledge of staff duties, knowledge of treatment techniques. When such knowledge is inappropriately located in the organization (i.e., patients' knowledge is as good as or better than staff's), the legitimacy of authority and control by staff is put in question. For example, if a patient has the same quality and quantity of information as ward staff, other patients may just as well bring their questions and problems to knowledgeable patients as to staff.

In the caste-type structure of the hospital, formal rewards are removed from the interaction system. In the interaction system, informal rewards from upper-status persons to lower-status persons are generally in the form of releasing public or private symbols (i.e., information). We shall try to show that informal rewards in terms of symbol distribution result in the rearrangement of social distance patterns and the consequent status and power threats. Let us now turn to a discussion of the three sociometric status groups in terms of the consequences of their contact patterns for the problems under consideration.

Hi Positives. Patients who received the most choices as desirable roommates also had relatively little contact with staff (see Table 4-1), and what contacts they did have were concentrated in non-troublesome areas. In a very real sense, these are patients "who know their place in the system." Because they are on good terms with both staff and patients, they become very desirable roommate choices. A "Hi Positive" will not balk at staff orders and ward routine. If she were to resist a ward rule to scrub the floor once a week, this would either throw the entire burden on the roommate or, probably, implicate the roommate as a troublemaker.

The "Hi Positive" spends most of her time in interaction with other patients and willingly supports and acts out norms of privacy and exchange, thus enhancing her popularity. Her limited contact with staff also enhances her "good patient" identity and makes her even more desirable as a friend.

Hi Negatives. The "Hi Negatives" stand out for their relatively frequent contact with staff as well as for the amount of contact that involves doing favors for staff. They have adopted a conversion mode of adaptation and maintain strong identification with the staff. The rejection of these patients by other patients is not simply the result of doing favors for staff or being closely identified with them, but is primarily due to their attempt to maximize social distance from other patients and minimize social distance from staff.[12] Let us illustrate this point:

Hi Negatives do a great many favors for staff. They run errands, do ward chores, and convey information. The staff becomes quite dependent on their help and information. They make the job of the attendant much easier in many ways, so that attendants must reward these patients. One salient feature of the reward structure is *contact with* or *access to* higher-status persons. Thus, attendants allow Hi Negatives to sit in the nurses' office or "hang around" at the office door. In the process, these patients attempt to stop being patients by engaging in equal-status interaction. The use of the first name or nickname variations on the last name is frequently attempted.[13]

[12] The direction of the causal process we are outlining requires additional comment. The general model indicates that relations with subordinates are a function of relationships with superordinates. It was found that attendants who were able to minimize distance from superordinates did not maximize distance from subordinates, while attendants who were unable to minimize distance from superordinates did maximize distance from subordinates. Three levels in the organization (i.e., the actor, his superordinate, and his subordinate) are needed to test the model, but in the present context we are dealing with data from only two levels (attendants and patients), so that our causal sequence is not too clear. What we are suggesting in this section, is that Hi Negatives seek to maximize distance from other patients and minimize distance from staff.

[13] Contact with attendants can, of course, mean something more than simply gaining access to public and private symbols. Such contacts may provide the patient with privacy, special privileges, and access to material goods.

Even more important is the fact that these patients seek equal-status contact with persons of *higher* status than the ward attendants. Thus the status threat is not only in having access to the private symbols of ward attendants but also in having access to the private symbols of persons of higher status than the attendants. The following exchange between the ward nurse and ward attendant illustrates the sensitivity of this situation.

ATTENDANT   Some of the patients here think they're smart the way they get chummy with the doctors and even the superintendent, calling them by their first names. The other patients don't like that, it really disgusts them.

NURSE   That's the same thing with Celine, isn't it? Since she went over on Companion Service all she talks about is Dr. Fields this and Dr. Fields that. How she had coffee with Dr. Fields, or how Dr. Fields got her a cup of coffee or gave her a cigarette, that's all you hear from her.

ATTENDANT   Well, you know his wife doesn't help matters either. Whenever she comes on the ward she stops to talk with Celine. Calls Celine by her first name and lets Celine call her by her first name. With things like that, it's no wonder we have trouble with these girls.

A similar incident with the same patient reveals the same type of staff response to a status threat.

ATTENDANT   [*to observer*] We really had a go-round with Celine yesterday. Friday she went over to Dr. Fields asking if she could go on Companion Service. Dr. Fields said she would have to talk to me about it. Well, Celine came back on the ward saying that Dr. Fields said it was O.K. for her to go on Companion Service. The other girls [patients] really got upset over this; they didn't know whether to believe her or not, but Celine kept saying it over and over and finally convinced them.
  Then Dr. Fields came on the ward yesterday and I told him what was going on. He cleared up what was actually said to Celine and said it was my ward and I should run it as I see fit. That's just the way I feel. I'll quit working if I have to take all that aggravation and trouble with the job. Anyway, Dr. Fields brought it up at Medical Staff yesterday, and Dr. Powell came back to me saying he heard I was unhappy about something. Well, I told him I was unhappy; that I thought she should be transferred to 14—that's where our "vegetables" are. But I can't work this ward without his support. He tried his old psychology on me, saying are you going to admit defeat and let Celine beat you. I told him yes, I know when I'm beaten and I'm not going to take anymore.
  They caused Celine to be that way. They let her call them by their first names. Mrs. Fields comes in here and falls all over Celine and lets her call her by her first name.

Dr. Powell asked me if I wanted him to talk to Celine. I said yes, that's your place to tell her. Well, he got her in here [nurses' office on the ward] and gave it to her. He told her about stepping all over the personnel, *moving in on everyone whenever they get the least bit friendly.* He told her we were washing our hands of trying to help her—we were all through. Why, you know, she really embarrassed Dr. Fields when she went to see him. He told me so.

Relations on the ward between the Hi Negatives and the ward attendants take on the appearance of a continual cycle. Whenever the patient becomes too "bold" in her contacts with attendants and poses a threat problem, she is deprived of contact with or access to the attendants. In staff language, they "sit on the patient." Free access to the nurses' office is denied, which means that the attendants must themselves wash medication glasses, clean up the office, and the like. All contacts between the attendants and the sanctioned patient become highly formalized—for example, each party makes a point of calling each other by Mrs. or Miss titles. This period of minimized contact and maximized social distance is short-lived, however. The attendant, confronted by the press of time in her essential duties, must seek help for housekeeping chores. Thus, the attendant allows the sanctioned patient to resume her former place on the ward and the cycle begins once again.

The following incident with another Hi Negative, Betty L., reveals the connection between dependence on these patients and the subsequent status threats.

(The attendants on Ward X were invited to a small birthday party for another attendant on Ward Y. The problem is that they are not to leave the ward unattended.)

MRS. TALBOT   What shall we do, take turns going over to have cake and coffee?

MRS. BENDER   No, why don't you have Betty L. watch the ward? You can depend on her to run things.

(They call in Betty L.)

MRS. TALBOT   We won't be gone very long. If anyone calls, tell them we'll call back because we're busy upstairs, and then call us at _____. Keep an eye on the girls so that they don't do anything they shouldn't.

It should be noted that Betty L. is not selected for her ability to get cooperation from other patients, but for her willingness to see that other patients do not do anything "wrong." In other words, while another patient might get greater cooperation from the patients, she would not have sufficient identification with the staff to keep her friends from coming into the nurses' office to look at their charts or take an extra supply of tobacco.

After returning from the birthday party, the two attendants thank Betty L. and compliment her on how she handled the ward. They then joke with her about the fact that maybe she should be the charge attendant on the ward.

Several days later, two administrative nurses from Nursing Service are in the nurses' office on Ward X discussing something with Mrs. Talbot. While they are talking, Betty L. opens the dutch door and walks right into the office. She walks between the seated nurses and Mrs. Talbot into the bathroom, where she gets a bucket, a mop, and soap suds. After getting her equipment, she leaves the office. Conversation between the staff during this time stops. They are all watching Betty L. This situation is really a marked violation of status barriers, for although a number of patients do enter the nurses' office without asking to get various things, they never enter when various administrative personnel not attached to the ward are in the office. After the nurses leave, Mrs. Talbot calls Betty L. into the office.

MRS. TALBOT   I don't know where you get the nerve to come in here like that; that was the height of rudeness, Betty. Don't you ever break in here again when the nurses are here. They come in here because they want to talk in private.

BETTY L.   [*angrily*] Well, I could tell you a few things about that. [*Walks out and slams door.*]

MRS. TALBOT   [*to observer*] That girl just wants to take over. She'll push herself right in if you give her half a chance.

These incidents illustrate what we mean by the statement that Hi Negatives pose a status threat to ward attendants. One interesting aspect of this situation is the chronic bind in which both the patients and the ward staff find themselves. The attendants' dependence on Hi Negatives for assistance on the ward is paid for with some loss of status. The patients, who are dependent on the attendants for status gains, through contacts, must pay for their gains by periodically accepting painful rebuffs by the staff and by being alienated from other patients.

It is precisely because of their alienation from other patients that these particular patients were most frequently chosen as undesirable roommates. As we suggested earlier, it was *not* because they were identified with staff or did favors for staff, but because they disassociated themselves from other patients. When the Hi Negatives interact with other patients they do so not as patients, but as representatives of staff. They usually repeat and enforce ward rules for other patients, or remind them of what Mrs. Talbot or Dr. Powell said about something or other. They try constantly to put other patients "in their place," and thus to maximize social distance between themselves and other patients. Hi Negatives criticize other patients for untidiness, uncleanliness, poor eating habits and table manners, and the like. If we could create a visual picture of the Hi Negatives in action, we would portray them as attempting to "reach up" to staff status by standing on the backs of other patients and "pushing down."

The pattern of "pushing down" members of one's own group as a way of moving up is interestingly demonstrated in the negative sociometric choices among the Hi Negatives; they made five of their eight possible negative choices among themselves. Thus, the patients who are negatively selected most frequently by all the patients are also negatively selected within their own sociometric group. These choices seem to reflect the general "pushing down" strategy of the Hi Negatives. Because they all compete for contact with and access to ward personnel, they also seek to "push down" their closest competitors.

Hi Negatives on Ward X organize their behavior on the ward in a way that minimizes social distance between themselves and staff and maximizes social distance between themselves and other patients. The former results in status threats to staff by the Hi Negatives, while the latter results in a persistent state of conflict with other patients.

Hi Leaders. The two patients most frequently chosen as potential leadership candidates on Ward X exhibit the highest overall contact ratio with ward attendants, and they show rather marked interaction in the areas of "Criticism" and "Formal Business" (see

Table 4-1). But Julia T. is high on "Criticism" while Nora P. is high on "Formal Business." This split in the type of contact pattern reveals an interesting feature of the leadership roles that emerge within the inmate world.

Nora P. is the formal leader on the ward. She is the elected ward president and the ward representative to the inter-ward council. Julia T., who holds no formal position on the ward, is clearly the informal leader. We shall try to show that the emergence of the informal leader is a response to the inevitable "conservatism" of the formal leader. Both leaders will be discussed in light of our contention that they pose a power threat to ward staff.

The Formal Leader. As the elected ward president, Nora P. is responsible for representing the patients to the staff. This includes channeling requests, complaints, suggestions, and the like to appropriate persons on the ward or in the hospital in general. As the ward representative to the inter-ward council she conveys information, complaints, and requests, which go beyond ward staff responsibilities, to the upper administrative staff. (Inter-ward council meetings are usually attended by the director of Nursing Services, nursing area supervisors, and on occasion, the clinical director and superintendent.) In addition, she brings information back to patients as well as *information, suggestions, and orders to ward staff.* The latter aspect is significant for the initiation of interaction and activity in unequal status relationships. Here a patient has control over information and distributes it to ward staff. *The ward president clearly represents an example of inappropriately located knowledge and sanctions.*

With respect to knowledge, the ward president has more contact with persons in the upper echelons of the hospital hierarchy than the average ward attendant could hope for. She hears various administrative staff express opinions on the hospital structure and operation that lower-level staff may never hear. Whenever the ward president returns from an inter-ward council meeting, she is faced with the probing questions of ward attendants: Who was there? What did you talk about? What did so and so say about that? The sensitivity of ward staff to inappropriately located knowledge is revealed in the following incident:

PATIENT [*standing at the door of nurses' office*] What are you going to do with all the extra room after some of the girls leave, Mrs. Talbot?

MRS. TALBOT No one's leaving here for a while yet, Celeste.

PATIENT Oh, yes, they are. Some of the girls are going to move over to another ward.

MRS. TALBOT Where did you get that idea from?

PATIENT Mrs. Small [administrative nurse] told me some of the girls here are going over to AB.

(*The patient leaves.* MRS. TALBOT *immediately calls the Nursing Service and inquires as to the reliability of a rumor concerning the transfer of patients to Ward AB.* MRS. TALBOT *is told there is a possibility of such a move, but gets no specific statement.*)

MRS. TALBOT [*to observer*] How do you like that? They never said anything to me. *I have to wait until a patient comes and tells me.* That puts me in an awful position. Now the other girls will start coming to me all upset over whether they're going to be transferred. What can I tell them? I've got to say *I don't know*—that's awful.

Turning to the inappropriate location of sanctions, we find this again in Nora P.'s access to upper echelons at inter-ward council meetings. Nora has at her command the power to decide what she will discuss at ward meetings, or what information from the ward she will convey to inter-ward council meetings. She can cast the ward staff in a very unfavorable light by repeated complaints regarding ward policies, ward situations, or ward staff. Similarly, Nora may make comments or suggestions that will flatter the ward staff or indicate the patients' satisfaction with the ward staff. For example, from time to time at inter-ward council meetings a representative will get up and say: "At our last ward meeting, we voted that Mrs. Green [ward attendant] should have a raise because she is such a good attendant." Everyone generally laughs at the suggestion, including the attending administrators, one of whom may reply, "There will be an extra ten dollars in her envelope this week." The full significance of the situation should not be lost in its humorous context. The attendant mentioned for the salary increase does not easily forget the incident and will often repeat it to other attendants, nurses, and doctors as a means of enhancing her position in the hospital.

However, although the formal leader on the ward does command a relatively powerful position, her orientation toward staff becomes increasingly conservative during her period of tenure. At first, the formal leader "processes" and transmits almost all patient complaints and comments. She is, at this time, truly representing the patients to the staff. With her increased contact with staff and with significant persons in the administration, she becomes much more sensitive to the kinds of complaints that are *appropriate* and the kinds that are *inappropriate*. Gradually, the formal leader evolves from a "champion for patients' rights," to a moderate who "understands the problems facing the staff." Quite realistically, the formal leader wishes to maintain her rather enviable position for the full period of her election. For although she has been elected, she could easily be removed by suggestions from the ward staff that she has a bad influence on the other patients and is overly negativistic or belligerent. The formal leader could not sow the seeds of discontent very long without being removed.

This "conservatism" does not reflect an identification with staff and an alienation from patients; it simply means that the formal leader has become less openly critical of the staff, staff procedures, and the hospital in general. This is the reason for the emergence of an informal leader on the ward. She may attack the hospital and the staff without risking any loss of status benefits, and in doing so actually enhance her status with respect to other patients.

The Informal Leader. Julia T. is reported to be the most troublesome patient on the ward. Ask any of the shift attendants which patient gives them the most trouble and this is the kind of response:

ATTENDANT   There's no trouble answering that one. Julia T., who else? She goes around here sassing everyone back, saying anything she wants, and what can we do about it—nothing! What she needs is to be treated the way she treats everyone else.

To fully understand the role of the informal leader, we shall examine her relations with other patients, and the nature of the criticism she directs toward staff. The informal leader's behavior in each of these areas indicates why she is accorded such high status by the patients.

In her relations with other patients, the informal leader is bound to no one in any enduring relationship. In general, her behavior on the ward violates one or another of the relatively shared patient norms. In her first contact with the observer, the informal leader used a number of tabooed words in describing herself and other patients.

JULIA T.   Are you one of the doctors here to help us nuts get better?
OBSERVER   No, I'm not a doctor.
JULIA T.   All the smart doctors come here to help us lunatics. Well, you better watch your step that you don't go "loony" like the rest of us.

Another incident reflects her willingness to attack other patients for what can be considered "acting like a patient."

(*Several patients are sitting out on the lounge smoking and talking. Julia walks in and sits down. The other patients are talking about jewelry and their boyfriends. After listening for a while, Julia starts to criticize them.*)

JULIA T.   Can't you do anything else but talk about jewelry and your boy-friends? You're always trying to connive jewelry out of someone. What good are all your earrings anyway? And your boyfriends, all they think about is "here's another rich bitch whose skirts I can get under." Who needs those alcoholics [*the boyfriends*] anyway. You always have to buy their coffee and cigarettes, don't you? I'd rather be with the "nuts" like me.

These are things the formal leader would never say. She maintains rather harmonious ties with most other patients. Why then should Julia T. receive so much support from the other patients? We would suggest that it is precisely because of her openly critical pose toward ward staff in particular and the hospital in general that she enjoys such high status. This is so in spite of her relatively deviant position with respect to patient norms.

In her criticism of staff, the informal leader becomes a means by which much of the latent aggression and hostility of other patients can be channeled and expressed. During ward rounds, for example, the informal leader usually tells a few "psychiatric jokes," for which she gets considerable support in the form of open laughter.

More important, however, is the way in which she comes to the defense of *any* patient against the ward staff. The following incident provides an excellent example.

(Lizzie S., one of the more disliked patients on the ward [a Hi Negative] has just returned from talking to two of the social workers handling her case. She tells the ward attendant what the social workers told her, and she is crying and upset at the same time. Julia T. is listening.)

LIZZIE S.   I told them I thought all my difficulty was in getting along with the other girls, especially Celine and Ruth *[two other Hi Negatives]*.

MRS. TALBOT   What did they tell you to do, Lizzie?

LIZZIE S.   Mr. _____ and Miss _____ said I shouldn't talk to either Ruth or Celine, and that I should stay away from the other girls too. They said I shouldn't speak to anyone else unless I'm spoken to.

MRS. TALBOT   That sounds like good advice to me. You'd better follow it.

JULIA T.   Good advice! What's the poor girl supposed to do with her tongue? I never heard of anything so stupid.

(JULIA walks into nurses' office and puts her arms around LIZZIE's shoulders and leads her out of the office and down the hall.)

JULIA T.   Come on, Lizzie. You go down now and relax and take a nap. You'll feel much better when you get up.

An important aspect of the informal leader's criticism of staff is that it is *not* merely a nonspecific hostility that manifests itself in any situation in which the staff may be criticized. Rather, she stays "on top of the staff" in relevant areas of organizational rules and procedures both on and off the ward. Julia T. prides herself in her knowledge of the hospital ("Why, Mrs. Talbot even has to ask me about things about this place. She doesn't know it as well as me"), for it is precisely on these grounds that she usually makes her attack. Thus, we return to our concern with the *power threat* that the Hi leaders pose to staff, through the mechanism of inappropriately located knowledge. An excellent example of this can be seen in the following "Bermuda shorts incident."

(Julia T. is walking from her room to the dayroom. She is wearing Bermuda shorts. Mrs. Rand, the ward nurse, calls Julia over.)

MRS. RAND   All right, Julia, off with the shorts; you know that you girls are not allowed to wear them.

JULIA T.   What do you mean? We were allowed to wear them last year. It was always O.K.

MRS. RAND   Well, I'm telling you it's not O.K. So take them off, please.

JULIA T.   I'm not taking them off because I know we're allowed to wear them, and I'll prove it.

(JULIA T. *goes over to Nursing Service and returns in a few minutes with two administrative nurses,* MRS. SANDS *and* MRS. CROWELL. *They walk into the nurses' office where* MRS. RAND, *the ward nurse, and* MRS. TALBOT, *the ward attendant, are seated.* JULIA T. *remains at the dutch door.*)

MRS. SANDS   [*to* MRS. RAND] Julia said you wouldn't let her wear shorts, and she said the patients have always been allowed to wear them. Mr. West [*director of Nursing Service*] wasn't in so I couldn't check on what the rule is.

MRS. RAND   I remember a Nursing Service memo stating that shorts were not to be worn by patients. As a matter of fact, there is also a rule against staff wearing shorts on the hospital grounds.

MRS. SANDS   Did you tell her she couldn't wear shorts ever, or just in certain places?

MRS. RAND   [*slightly angry*] I just followed Mr. West's memo.

JULIA T.   [*steps in the office from the door*] The memo that came through last summer said we couldn't wear short shorts, but that Bermudas were O.K.

MRS. CROWELL   [*to* MRS. TALBOT] Why don't you look through the old memos [*in the ward memo book*] and see if you can find anything.

(*After five minutes or so,* MRS. TALBOT *comes up with a memo regarding summer apparel for patients. She reads aloud of a line in the memo stating:* ". . . *shorts may be worn, provided they are a decent length above the knee.*")

JULIA T.   See, I told you!

(MRS. RAND *gets into an involved discussion with the two administrative nurses concerning what constitutes* "*a decent length above the knee.*" *They finally agree that the wording is ambiguous, since the length of shorts above the knee would vary with different anatomical structures.*)

MRS. RAND   I'm sure there was another order. I don't know, though, they change them so fast.

MRS. SANDS   I'll check with Mr. West for sure, and call you back.

(*The two administrative nurses leave; the ward nurse leaves shortly after. About fifteen minutes later, there is a phone call for* MRS. RAND *stating that Bermudas are appropriate summer apparel for patients.*)

MRS. TALBOT   [*to observer*] Poor Mrs. Rand, she really got stepped on. You have to watch your step with that Julia, she usually knows what she's talking about.

We indicated, with the formal leader, that the power threat was primarily related to inappropriately located sanctions (as well as knowledge). With the informal leader, on the other hand, a large reservoir of inappropriately located knowledge is combined with a rather militant orientation toward the staff. This combination gives the informal leader power to influence and control the behavior of many of the other patients.

This, then, is the nature of the power threat posed by the informal leader to the ward staff.[14] Some latent consequences of the informal leader's behavior, however, appear to have certain stabilizing effects upon the operation of the ward. As we have already indicated, the informal leader provides a convenient channel for expressing many of the other patients' latent hostilities. In a sense, she can "act out" for everyone else. In addition, the informal leader performs the same function for the ward staff. In her attacks upon the ward psychiatrist, for example, she can express many of the feelings of the ward attendants. This is quite evident in the subtle support she receives from ward attendants whenever she tells one of her "psychiatrist jokes." Similarly, the "Bermuda shorts incident" helped take the ward nurse "down a peg," which

---

[14] It is interesting to note the apparent awareness the informal leader has of the fact that she is playing a part (i.e., role) which has been externally thrust upon her, and which is most difficult to leave. Following are some selected comments from an interview with the informal leader which are illustrative of this point.

Q.   Do you usually follow the doctor's advice?

A.   No! Well, I should say I try, but I usually do it secretly without the rest of the girls knowing it.

Q.   Why do you do that?

A.   Oh, it's natural. You're fighting for a little respect—it's like in a factory when your boss does something for you, you have to worry about the other employees.

Q.   How do you get along with your doctor?

A.   We usually battle. It's hard. What he doesn't know is that I really try to respect him, but I can't. It seems like he won't let me forget all the rotten things I've said about him in the past.

the ward attendant cannot do so blatantly. Thus, though the ward attendant may be the object of the informal leader's attacks *some of the time,* others in the hospital hierarchy will be the object at other times.

Another positive function of the informal leader is that she continually sets the boundaries for appropriate behavior on the ward. She tests the utility of existing rules and initiates action for the emergence of new rules. It is perhaps paradoxical that through the patients' leaders information from a number of levels in the hospital should be made available to the ward personnel. Ward attendants, by the nature of their jobs, have limited access to other levels in the hospital hierarchy. Their information comes in the form of specific directives from Nursing Service, or brief contacts with the ward physician. The ward leaders, on the other hand, have considerable freedom of movement and access to persons variously located in the hospital hierarchy. With this access comes information regarding a variety of organizational rules, procedures, and the like. For example, in their contacts with other patients the ward leaders gather considerable information about the way things are done on other wards. Through the ward leaders, information is collected and coordinated more effectively than would be possible through the ward attendants alone.

STAFF REACTIONS TO STATUS THREATS AND POWER THREATS

We have indicated above that the Hi Positives are primarily involved in harmonious relationships with other patients, and in limited nonthreatening contact with staff. Hi Negatives pose a status threat to staff by continually seeking to minimize social distance with the staff. Hi Leaders do not attempt to minimize social distance, but rather attempt to adjust power relations through the control of sanctions and information.

Although much of our material illustrates staff reactions to these three groups of patients, we would like to look at staff reactions specifically in the area of maintaining social distance. For example, if what we have said about the behavior of the three patient groups has any validity, we would expect the ward staff to be primarily concerned with maximizing social distance with the Hi Negatives.

We would not expect this with the Hi Leaders because their attacks are not directed toward ward staff specifically, but are generalized to hospital rules and procedures and directed to a variety of staff status positions.

In order to examine staff reactions to the three patient groups, we asked ward attendants to rate how well the patients are characterized by fifteen statements which describe different attitudes and behavior of mental patients. The statements were also rated by members of the medical staff on how well they describe a hypothetical patient who is well enough for a discharge. The difference between attendants' ratings of the three patient groups and medical staff's rating of the hypothetically "well" patient is taken as a measure of "deviations from normality." The more a patient "deviates" from the hypothetically well patient, the "sicker" that patient is being labeled by ward attendants. We also assume that the definition of patient as "sick" is a means of maintaining social distance from that patient.

An analysis of the attendants' ratings indicates that they attribute to the Hi Negatives the largest deviations from normality; we interpret this as attendants' effort to maximize social distance from those patients who make the greatest efforts to minimize social distance. The ratings of "deviations from normality" for both the Hi Leaders and Hi Positives are similar and much lower than the ratings for the Hi Negatives. These findings, therefore, are consistent with our earlier discussion about patient threats and staff reactions.

Thus, we have isolated in this chapter what we might call a *paradox of organizational outcomes*. Let us assume, for example, that one of the goals of the mental hospital is to provide for a primary type of contact between patients and attendants. This goal is pursued for the general purpose of resocialization (i.e., the transmission of staff values and appropriate standards of behavior), which takes place primarily through the process of social interaction. We can see from this chapter, however, that a considerable amount of social interaction is generally accompanied by certain types of violation of status barriers (such as status threats and power threats). As a result, the goal of patient contact with upper-level staff can be attained only at the risk of violating a status barrier and making advances on the "staff world." Achieving primary-type contact with staff, which is designed to aid the therapeutic process, actually operates to the disadvantage of the patient because she is tagged with the label of "troublemaker" or "pushy." On the other hand, the patient who has a minimum amount of contact with staff, and thereby earns the title of "a good patient," does so at the expense of losing the potentially beneficial consequences of primary relationships with staff.

If the objectives of the hospital were truly to resocialize, rehabilitate, and release patients, then those who achieved close relationships with staff would not become a threat, because attainment of social closeness would either precede or be predictive of a discharge.

In the next chapter we shall try to demonstrate the ways in which the social distance strategies among patients and staff described in this chapter influence relationships among hospital staff.

5

Social Distance,
Bureaucratic Authority,
and Therapeutic Relationships

Being on a mental hospital ward after dark is a very different experience from daytime duty for staff. Ward doors are locked, all patients are back on the ward, and the number of staff persons on the ward and in the hospital in general is sharply reduced. Doctors return to their homes, with one of them being "on call" if needed. Nurses do not work nights, except for one who remains in the executive building and is "on call" as the senior person in authority. The number of attendants who work the night shifts is also reduced so that open wards have only a single attendant on duty.

Although patients' feelings about hospital life at night are hard to acertain, there is evidence that ward staff tend to feel "cut off" and somewhat vulnerable to unknown and poorly articulated fears at this time. The nurses' office, the place patients seek contact with staff during the day, becomes a refuge for the attendant at night. It is difficult for him or her to avoid the feeling of being a "prisoner" surrounded by fifty-odd patients whom he does not really know.

The feeling of being isolated, without the social support of colleagues, and in an atmosphere of some anxiety, if not outright fear, is a reality that must be dealt with by the night-shift attendant. The night attendant faces a special problem of maintaining social control on the ward without the support of all the trappings of authority that are found on the day shift. He also faces the problem of determining the scope of his authority, which is ambiguous at night because of the absence of other authority figures.

In the previous chapter we focused attention on the way patients responded to the formal hospital structure and modified it through their own efforts to engage in meaningful and self-enhancing social relationships. In this chapter we shall shift our attention to the hospital staff, who share with patients the problem of developing and maintaining a favorable self-concept and a desirable position in the hospital social structure.

We shall compare the day and night shifts on Ward X in terms of formal authority relationships between staff and between patients and staff. The specific focus of attention is the extent to which day and night attendants adhere to and comply with organizational rules and directives of physicians. We shall maintain the view of an organization, developed in the previous chapter, as being a network of social distance patterns built about a set of fixed positions, whose occupants behave so as to maintain or enhance their status in the hierarchy. More specifically, it is suggested that attendants who are able to minimize social distance between themselves and doctors are less likely to maximize social distance between themselves and patients.

In their study of a small private psychiatric hospital, Stanton and Schwartz recognized the close connection between the way attendants are treated, and the way they, in turn, treat patients:

. . . if personnel are treated harshly and in an authoritarian manner, if they are ordered about without concern for them as persons, if decisions are made arbitrarily and their opinions are neither asked nor respected, the probability is high that they will use similar approaches to the patients. It will be difficult for them to contribute to the patient's self-esteem when their own is under attack.[1]

Work Shifts and Compliance with Rules and Directives

The work routine in the hospital is organized around the day shift (8:00 A.M. to 4:00 P.M.), the evening shift (4:00 to midnight), and the night shift (midnight to 8:00 A.M.). Attention here is focused upon the day and evening shifts.[2]

[1] Alfred H. Stanton and Morris S. Schwartz, *The Mental Hospital* (New York: Basic Books, Inc., 1954), p. 61.

[2] The midnight to 8:00 A.M. shift is not analyzed because of the completely different character of life on this shift. The patients are already in bed, and the attendant may have little contact with any except the oc-

The *day shift* is the period of greatest activity for both patients and staff. On open wards, patients work, go to daily activities, and move on and off the ward with great frequency. For the staff, the day shift provides the greatest amount of contact among doctors, nurses, attendants, and other adjunct therapists. For the attendants, in particular, there are more occasions for contact with the ward nurse and ward physician than on any of the other shifts.

The most important feature of the *evening shift* is the fact that the number of personnel on the wards is greatly reduced. The attendants have little contact with physicians and nurses and only limited contact with other attendants. (Although Ward X has two attendants on the evening shift, many wards have only one.) While staff life decreases on the evening shift, the tempo of patient life on the ward increases. Working patients are back on the ward, alternative activities are limited, and, after a certain time, the ward doors are locked and patients must remain on the ward. With the increased density of the patient population come increased occasions for patient-patient and patient-staff contact. Arguments and fights are more frequent, and they tend to become magnified, with the increased likelihood that dissatisfactions will be transmitted from patient to patient. The safety valve of the open door and alternative activities cannot operate to mitigate strained situations.

The allocation of attendants to positions in the hospital, whether on ward assignments or shift assignments, does not seem to follow a procedure that would result in "fitting" particular personality types to particular work assignments. In fact, the informal hospital policy on work assignments is designed to avoid such a tendency. A top administrator in the hospital pointed out in an interview that work assignments are periodically rotated for the expressed purpose of avoiding a tendency for attendants to "get too comfortable on a ward."

The two day-shift and two evening-shift attendants on Ward X were found to be markedly different with respect to their following

---

casional problem sleeper or actively disturbed patient. Moreover, whatever problems do emerge are usually individual rather than collective in nature. They are not likely to involve a fight or an argument between two patients, or a situation of mood contagion. Thus, the attendant on this shift is relatively protected from a variety of threatening situations that could develop in the patient population.

of organizational rules, or behavior in accordance with the directives of a superordinate.

On the evening shift, attendants continually manifest great concern with following hospital rules. Patient requests for various things are evaluated in terms of established procedures. Evening attendants will not interpret and act upon a slightly unclear or ambiguous memo but will leave it for further clarification—usually for the day shift. One indication of this greater concern over adherence to rules is observed during the change in shifts. When the evening attendant takes over the ward and the symbolic transfer of keys is made, she will with maximum predictability immediately lock the medication cabinet. Although it should, according to hospital rules, be locked at all times, it is always open during the day shift.

In many other respects the behavior of the day attendants stands in sharp contrast to that of the evening attendants. The day attendants sometimes give medication without the permission of the ward physician. They often allow patients to keep money received in the mail rather than turn it in to their canteen funds as required by the rules. The ward physician's order that a certain patient should not have her dolls to play with is ignored in favor of the attendant's opinion that "her dolls help her more than they hurt her."

Interviews with the two day attendants and two evening attendants supported these observations. Each attendant was asked, first, to respond to eight pairs of items which refer to the degree of formality of her relationships with the ward physician (one item in each pair indicating high formality and the other low formality);[3] and, second, to indicate her opinions concerning the need for greater clarity of thirteen hospital rules governing the care and treatment of patients.[4]

[3] Examples of pairs of these items are the following descriptions of the doctor:

a. He sticks closely to procedure.
a. He is less worried about procedure and more willing to make reasonable exceptions.
b. He really knows procedure cold.
b. He is not too interested in knowing every rule in the book.

[4] The rules covered patients' sexual relationships, appropriate clothing for patients, hours and limits, food on the ward, private property, and the like.

With respect to the degree of formality in attendant-physician relationships, both of the day attendants selected all eight statements that were descriptive of low formality with the physician, while one evening attendant selected six of eight high-formality statements and the other selected five. With respect to the need for clarity of hospital rules, both day attendants indicated a need for "much clarification" on two of the thirteen rules, while both evening attendants indicated a need for "much clarification" on nine.[5]

These data obtained from both observation and interviewing of attendants are quite consistent with the findings of Segal, whose investigations showed night-shift nurses to be more custodial and rule-oriented in their attitudes toward patients.[6] Why is it, then, that the day attendant behaves considerably less in accord with formal organizational directives than does the evening attendant? Similarly, why, in the almost complete absence of formal supervision, is the evening attendant more concerned with following and enforcing formal rules? I shall attempt to explain these differences by an examination of the social structure on the day and evening shifts.

In looking for the sources of the day attendant's less compliant behavior and attitude toward rules and directives, the exchange system on the ward will be examined first; second, the bargaining power of the day attendant; and third, the "team approach" to treatment. These will be viewed as links in a process leading to a decrease in social distance between the attendant and the physician and a corresponding breakdown of authority patterns.

THE EXCHANGE SYSTEM

Other studies have stressed the importance that contact with high-status persons has for low-status persons in the hospital caste hier-

[5] The possibility may be raised that these observed behavioral and attitudinal differences are due to individual rather than structural differences. However, questionnaire returns from 69 day attendants and 50 evening attendants bore out the tendency of the day attendants to express less need for clarification of the thirteen rules than was expressed by evening attendants.

[6] Bernard E. Segal, "Nurses and Patients: Time, Place and Distance," *Social Problems,* 9 (1962), 257–64.

archy.[7] Such contacts, of a particular kind, are viewed as substitutes for promotion in a structure that does not provide for internal mobility. The attendant, for example, looks favorably upon the possibility of interaction with the ward physician. However, these desirable contacts do not come easily. To achieve them, the ward attendant utilizes two strategies: to "push down" others who are competing for status-enhancing contacts, and to make available to the physician behavior that is *over and above* the formally prescribed expectations for attendants. The former point is illustrated in the critical comments that attendants often make about the performance of their peers when speaking to the ward nurse or doctor.

The second strategy—behavior over and above the call of duty—is what the attendant "gives" to the physician with the expectation of certain returns such as contact, attention, and decrease in social distance. There is much that the attendant can "give" in this situation, inasmuch as the "rights" of the status-position attendant are the "duties" of the status-position doctor. What the attendant gives is flexibility regarding her status "rights," or willingness to perform the doctor's "duties" herself. For example, the ward doctor is required to make at least one daily visit to the ward, but his workload sometimes makes this almost impossible. In this situation the attendant can attempt to make her ward's needs more important than those of other wards and "insist" upon a ward visit, or she can accommodate herself to the physician's desires. This does not mean that the attendant is happy about the situation, for this "giving" creates problems for her in the performance of her duties. Consider the following comment by the day attendant regarding the doctor's failure to make ward rounds:

That's not right. He hasn't been here for over a week. He's been over on Sixteen two days in a row. Why doesn't he make a schedule that's fair to all the wards? The girls want to see him, and *I don't know how long I can hold them off.*

Thus the attendant withholds her demands on the physician and takes the burden of the complaining patients upon herself. In addition, even when the physician does make his regular ward visit the

[7] Leonard I. Pearlin and Morris Rosenberg, "Nurse-Patient Social Distance and the Structural Context of a Mental Hospital," *American Sociological Review,* 27 (February 1962), 56–65.

attendant can give "that something extra" by screening patient requests and by limiting the number of patients who see the physician.
Again, the attendant helps the physician at her own expense. For
while the physician is spared the additional work, the attendant
must face the disgruntled patients whom she has discouraged from
seeing the doctor.

In addition to foregoing the "rights" attached to her position, the
attendant may also perform "duties" that are formally the responsibility of the doctor. The duties usually involve the administrative
tasks that physicians must perform, but which they view with great
distaste. For example, the physician is required to rewrite medication orders for each patient at the beginning of each month—a
major task when several hundred patients are involved, but one
specifically assigned to the physician, who is expected to reevaluate
each patient's medication order and either increase, decrease, change,
or continue the medication. The ward attendant, who is quite sensitive to the physician's likes and dislikes, will rewrite the orders for
her ward and thereby obligate the physician for a returned favor.

This description of the exchange system on the ward may make
it seem rather one-sided, with the attendant on the short end of the
deal as she assists the physician beyond the formal expectations for
her position and, in doing so, makes her job much more difficult.
But the importance of what she receives in this exchange cannot be
underestimated. Contact with the physician, with its fringe benefits
of status enhancement, has considerable symbolic meaning for her.
This is evident whenever attendants get together and play their informal "can-you-top-this" game. Each attendant tells an incident
that indicates either how dependent the doctor is on her, how
often he compliments her work, how they talk informally about
personal or family matters, or how they talk informally about hospital matters. By such evidence of contact with upper-level staff, the
attendants seek to increase their informal position—their prestige
—in the hierarchy.

One can see in the attendants' desire for status-enhancing contacts the same motives that led patients to criticize their peers and
seek contact with higher-level staff. Both have little opportunity to
change their formal position in the hospital structure and both are
seeking evidence for, or validation of, their worth as persons or employees. Both attendants and patients, moreover, have little basis

for believing that how they spend their days "makes a difference," either as to whether they will ever get out of the hospital (for patients), or whether they have helped anyone else to get out (for attendants).

BARGAINING POWER

The attendant attains bargaining power when she can enlist the cooperation of the physician to enhance her own status within the hospital. In the initial stage of the unequal exchange she is without bargaining power, because she is only receiving access to, or contact with, the physician *without his active participation* in her status enhancement. However, as the unequal exchange relationship develops, the physician builds up a backlog of unpaid obligations which affect the formality of his relationship with the attendant. He must show some awareness of the principle of reciprocity and of the obligations and debts he has incurred in his relationship with the attendant—debts that can be repaid by enhancing her status.

The unequal exchange develops into a position of power for the attendant also because of the physician's dependence upon her as a person, and not as an occupant of a position. One of the basic tenets of a bureaucratic structure is that persons are replaceable as long as the positions remain. Thus, the removal of a person from a position in no way impairs the smooth operation of the organization, because a replacement assumes the set of duties attached to the position. However, in the interaction between the doctor and the day attendant on the study ward, the attendant, Mrs. Talbot, was nonreplaceable. The doctor was able to operate on the ward *to the extent* that Mrs. Talbot continued to make available to him a kind of behavior that was *over and above* the formal role requirements. The following is an example of the way in which the doctor's effectiveness on the ward was impaired when Mrs. Talbot was not around to assist him.

Mrs. Talbot has called in sick, and is replaced by Mrs. Nemar, who is not a regular attendant on any ward, but works as a relief attendant. This means that she never gets an opportunity to work closely and establish "ground rules" for appropriate behavior with any single physician. Dr. Powell is making the ward rounds with

Mrs. Nemar in attendance. He has already seen two patients in the nurses' office.

MRS. NEMAR   Lizzie S. is also waiting to see you, Doctor.

DR. POWELL   Well, I don't particularly want to see her. What does she want?

MRS. NEMAR   I don't know. All I know is that she said she wants to see you.

DR. POWELL   [*in a very deliberate, disciplining tone*] Mrs. Nemar, it's your job to screen these requests and handle those things you can yourself. You're here to protect me against just such situations.

A few moments later, Mrs. Nemar is reading one of the patient's charts which contains a medical order suggesting periodic checks on the patient's temperature.

MRS. NEMAR   I have to take a patient's temperature, is that all right?

DR. POWELL   Yes, fine.

MRS. NEMAR   When shall I take it?

DR. POWELL   Whenever you want.

MRS. NEMAR   How about twice a day, at 11:00 and 7:00?

DR. POWELL   You decide that for yourself.

MRS. NEMAR   Me! That's for you to decide; I can't make those decisions.

DR. POWELL   Well, I'm sorry, but you've got to decide some of these things for yourself.

This painful exchange is followed in a few moments by the ringing of the office phone. Dr. Powell is sitting at the desk, and a few inches from the phone. Mrs. Nemar is at the other end of the office, some fifteen feet from the phone. What Mrs. Nemar doesn't know is that Mrs. Talbot, the regular day attendant, always answers the phone when Dr. Powell is present. This is done as protection for Dr. Powell, who is given the option of "being there" or "not being there." After the phone rings several times, Dr. Powell picks up the phone and holds it up in the air in the direction of Mrs. Nemar. He does this without looking up from a patient's chart he is reading. Mrs. Nemar, who has not looked in the direction of the desk and doctor, is unaware that he is holding the phone for her to take, and walks out of the office into the dayroom. Dr. Powell finally looks up and sees Mrs. Nemar leaving the office. He answers the call himself. The area supervisor from Nursing Service is calling for Mrs. Nemar.

Dr. Powell yells very loudly and sarcastically: "Mrs. Nemar, would it be too much trouble for you to answer the phone?" Mrs. Nemar comes into the office, but before she takes the phone, Dr. Powell speaks to the area supervisor in a joking tone: "You have to watch her; this girl will do anything to get out of work."

These three incidents, which all took place within the span of the approximately forty minutes spent by the doctor on ward rounds, indicate the nature of his dependence upon the regular day attendant. She can use this dependence, and her backlog of unpaid obligations, in her bargaining for certain types of status-enhancing contacts. The following examples indicate the attendant's expectations regarding extra rewards *and her threat of withdrawal of cooperation* when such rewards are not forthcoming.

The day attendant, Mrs. Talbot, and the observer are discussing Dr. Kirk, the psychologist who handles group therapy with patients on Ward X.

MRS. TALBOT   One day he called me and asked me to help him start another therapy group by drawing up a list of girls who might get something from therapy. Strictly speaking, that's not my job. The ward doctor's supposed to do that. Well, I said I'd do it, and it took me some time. I had to check the girls' folders to see who had been in group therapy before and see if there were any specific orders against therapy. Anyway, I drew up a list and sent it over to him. Do you think he even as much as picked up the phone to say "Thank you"? No, sir, *he never said a word to me or the doctor about it.*

The other thing is that the girls don't like to go to his therapy sessions. They say the awfulest things about him, like he's stupid. The problem is that he's so cold. He won't say anything. One day I brought the girls over [*to therapy*], and when he walked in, he walked in right by me like a zombie. Didn't look at me or say hello. The girls just looked at me, and I looked at them. Well, I have to be careful what I say about him in front of the girls. If I was to say he was a ninny or something, none of the girls would ever go back again.

A second incident involved a discussion between the observer and Mrs. Talbot of the differences among doctors in the hospital and their relationship to attendants.

MRS. TALBOT   Well, some doctors will ask you for help in making decisions. Dr. Powell [*the ward doctor*] does that a lot. But take Dr. Hill; he wouldn't ask you anything or allow you to do anything on your own.

What they don't realize is that it only hurts them. When I worked under Dr. Brumel, I never really liked him. He would always be snapping orders and telling you what to do, as if he was saying, "I know everything and I don't need your help." He was always prescribing medications that no one knew anything about. The cabinet would be full of certain medications for a particular problem, but he would go ahead and order something completely new. *The thing is, that we never gave him our best. Instead, we had to hold back and be reserved. But that's what he asked for, they make you hold back and not give your best.*

These incidents reflect a shift in the locus of power on the ward, with the day attendant being able to exert considerable control over the ward physician. She is able to exchange her continued cooperation for such rewards as the physician's support in conflicts with other attendants or with nurses, his "advertising" her as an excellent attendant, and a decrease in social distance from him. The examples above indicate the attendant's reaction when rewards or payoffs are not received from the higher staff person.

THE TEAM APPROACH TO TREATMENT

The team approach to psychiatric treatment, in its most extreme form, is an expression of democratic social relationships. Staff members of varying status positions are thought to combine their treatment efforts in accordance with a single plan of procedure.[8] The

---

[8] The formal members of the psychiatric team on Ward X include the ward physician, the ward nurse, the ward attendant, the social worker assigned to the ward, and the work therapist assigned to the ward. In practice, the team generally consists of the physician, nurse, and attendant. Thus, at weekly ward rounds all members of the team will go, in a group, from patient to patient in the dayroom. Any or all members of the team ask or answer questions concerning a particular patient. After ward rounds, the team returns to the nurses' office and attempts to evaluate the accomplishments of ward rounds for that day. New programs for a particular patient, such as a new work assignment or a new approach to milieu therapy, are also discussed. No team member is supposed to make a unilateral decision concerning any aspect of a patient's program in the hospital. For example, the work therapist does not assign a patient to a new job without first consulting the other members involved.

expected advantages of the team approach are that (1) patients are not subjected to differing sets of expectations regarding appropriate behavior; (2) essential information concerning patients is more effectively communicated by persons working together; (3) specialized treatments offered by different staff may be coordinated so as to eliminate internal contradictions; and (4) the more staff who are concerned with a patient's treatment, the more information is available, and the more effective decisions regarding his treatment can be made. In addition to these patient-oriented advantages, there are advantages for the staff members involved. Staff members, especially lower staff, are thought to achieve greater commitment to their work by being a part of the therapeutic function of the hospital, rather than performing only its custodial function. This approach is also thought to produce more conscientious cooperation among lower staff in aiding the professional staff.

Certain informal norms emerge governing behavior among the team members. For one thing, team members are urged to contribute their ideas in the discussions. It might be assumed that in such discussions the higher the participant's status, the more contributions he would make to group discussions.[9] On the study ward, however, the greatest amount of information on any particular patient was usually provided by the day attendant. The ward physician might make the most insightful remarks and might summarize the discussion, but the ward attendant usually talked more than any other team member.

A second feature of the team approach is that disagreement and criticism are encouraged. Team members are expected to examine their own motives, as well as the motives of others, in their comments regarding patients. The approach is, for example: If you dislike a particular patient, don't hide it, but use it as a means to understand your own motives. Is she a threat to you? Why is she a threat to you? Are you responding as a professional person, or as a mother, or husband, or wife would? Thus, the situation is defined as legitimately allowing low-status persons to question, probe, or criticize the opinions and behavior of high-status persons. This is

[9] The relevance of this point in a psychiatric setting is made most cogently by William Caudill in *The Psychiatric Hospital as a Small Society* (Cambridge, Mass.: Harvard University Press, 1958), Chapter 10.

different from the office Christmas party, when the clerk may legitimately tell the boss what he thinks of him, for it is a legitimation of status violations that takes place not just once a year, but within the everyday work tasks of the persons involved.

The ward physician is the member of the team most likely to turn the discussion to an analysis of motives. He uses this technique primarily as a teaching device for other members of the ward team—so they, in turn, will be able to see their own behavior with patients in a more meaningful framework. He may often use other team members as examples, but he primarily uses situations involving himself. Thus, he discusses personal aspects of his own life, such as early childhood experiences, or his role as a husband or parent, to help the ward staff to understand the dynamics of a patient's behavior; and he also discusses his own professional insecurities—"I really don't know what I'm doing with Dora"—and his problems in dealing with patients—"I know I've rejected Ruth, but I can't stand that girl and I can't help it."

Such an approach may be quite useful in terms of the ultimate effectiveness of a psychiatric team, but it is probably antithetical to maintaining formal status barriers. It provides a situation of status exposure in which the attendant may have a feeling of oneness with the physician—a feeling based upon presumed shared insecurities, shared deficiencies in knowledge, and equal responsibility for the patients and the ward. Given this situation, the maintenance of social distance between formal positions becomes most difficult. The physician has made himself vulnerable to the lower staff by providing them with too much information regarding himself personally, and his formal position. As was suggested in Chapter Four, this may be viewed as a situation of inappropriate location of public and private knowledge which provides the lower-status person with a basis for crossing status lines.

Thus, three elements of the day shift—the exchange system, bargaining power, and the team approach—appear to be the main factors leading to the less rule-oriented behavior of the day attendant. Each element tends to decrease social distance between the physician and the attendant, or to provide the attendant with a basis for questioning the authority of the physician. It may be added that authority based upon expertise is very likely to be unstable, unless the expertise is demonstrated.[10] The large state mental hospital does not provide the physician with much of an opportunity to demonstrate the utility of his knowledge or to validate his ability to "heal." Given this situation, which is beyond the control of the physician, the existence of formal social-distance patterns would seem to be essential for the maintenance of his authority. However, on Ward X, the distance patterns are under constant attack, and one of the commodities the physician can exchange for cooperation is his social distance. This is not, of course, to say that personal qualities of the doctor may not also promote cooperation.[11]

THE EVENING SHIFT

None of the elements discussed above is relevant for evening attendants. They have little or no contact with the ward physician; thus, there is neither a system of exchange nor any bargaining power to be gained by the attendants. The evening attendants make such remarks as, "I hardly ever see the doctor," or "What team approach? No one has ever asked for my opinion about a patient." The evening attendant perceives the physician as formal in his approach, for what contact she has with him is usually through written messages, either from him directly or given orally by him to the day attendant, who in turn leaves a note in the charts for the

[10] See, for example, Alvin W. Gouldner, *Patterns of Industrial Bureaucracy* (Glencoe, Ill.: Free Press, 1954); and William M. Evan and Morris Zelditch, Jr., "A Laboratory Experiment on Bureaucratic Authority," *American Sociological Review,* 26 (December 1961), 883–93.

[11] This raises an interesting question about the relationship between competence or ability and status. For example, Dr. Powell is considered by most hospital personnel, professional and nonprofessional alike, to be *both* the best-liked and most competent doctor. This view is expressed particularly by the attendants. Thus, because Dr. Powell is most willing to exchange decreased social distance for cooperation, one might ask whether his reputation of being "most competent" is an artifact of being "best-liked." On the other hand, being "best-liked" could be an artifact of being "most competent." For example, a person who feels quite secure regarding his own abilities may be less concerned with the potential status threat of decreasing social distance, and thus interact informally with lower-level staff.

evening attendant. This tends to impersonalize and formalize the nature of the contact between the evening attendant and the physician. Thus, while the day attendant may ask the physician a question and receive an answer which can be clarified by brief discussion, the evening attendant receives information by way of the directive, which is not softened by the interpersonal context.

An evening attendant made the following comment on how she received information from the doctor:

> I usually get *written orders* from the doctor through a note he will leave, or an *order* written in the chart. Sometimes the notes I find from the day shift tell me what the doctor said about something or other. When I get them this way [*through day attendants*] they're usually not too clear.

It is also interesting that the evening attendant receives orders from the physician when, in fact, he gave none. For example, he may make some comment to the day attendant about a patient or procedure. The day attendant, in transmitting this information, translates it into an order from the doctor. Thus, practically all of the evening attendant's contact with the physician is in the form of orders or formal directives. The following incident clearly reveals this process at work.

Mrs. Minton, the evening attendant, has written the following note on a patient, Lola P., who has been giving her some trouble.

EVENING NOTE: JULY 24

Patient disturbed, sassy and smart. Given impression that Dr. Powell said she could do as she pleased. Goes to ball games, without signing out. Tonight [she] signed out for garden and went to ball game. I went after her at 9:15 P.M. and she came back and signed the book for 8:30 P.M. She resented being made to sign again.

When Mrs. Talbot, the day attendant, reads this note she is critical of Mrs. Minton's failure to understand Lola P.'s particular problem. During the course of the day, Mrs. Talbot engages Dr. Powell in a conversation regarding Lola P., in which both agree that Lola has made considerable progress and should be treated with understanding. What Mrs. Minton does not know is that both Mrs. Talbot and Dr. Powell feel that Lola is well enough to go home but is being unjustifiably held at the hospital because of unsympathetic relatives. On the day following Mrs. Minton's notes,

Mrs. Talbot writes the following nursing note, with the obvious connotation of a reply:

MORNING NOTE: JULY 25

Patient is very good during the 8:00 A.M. to 4:30 P.M. shift. Came to office [today] and asked for the razor to shave. Was very warm and uncomfortable because of her obese condition. Patient is overweight and because of being uncomfortable is very short and irritable at times. Spoke with doctor about Lola. Patient is trying very hard to do what's right even in spite of her many disappointments of late. This patient's family has rejected her and will not cooperate with the institution for patient's release from the hospital. Patient is suffering with edema in her feet and legs. Doctor told patient she did not have to work but patient works part-time in peeling room.

Here the day attendant has translated her own opinions concerning the handling of Lola P. into a directive from the ward doctor. Thus, the evening attendant is subjected to the actual directives from the ward physician, plus the directives of the day attendant which are transmitted as the doctor's orders. The incident also illustrates the manner in which the day attendant uses the physician as supportive of her own particular views—an example of the earlier description of the strategies by which the day attendant uses the physician to run the ward as she sees fit.[12]

It has been indicated that the evening attendant, as compared to the day attendant, engages in predominantly rule-oriented behavior. Her perceived formality of relationships with the ward doctor, stemming from the peculiar nature of her communications with him, is a part of the reason but not the entire reason. Probably the main factor is the almost complete absence of social support for her behavior.

The day attendant has available what may be called numerous supportive subsystems, the most important of which is her relationship with the ward physician. The evening attendant, on the other hand, is almost completely isolated from these supportive subsystems. She has little or no contact with the ward physician or nurse. She rarely sees other attendants during her shift, and once the ward

[12] For additional evidence on the power of attendants see Thomas J. Scheff, "Control Over Policy by Attendants in a Mental Hospital," *Journal of Health and Human Behavior*, 2 (1961), 93–105; and David Mechanic, "Sources of Power of Lower Participants in Complex Organizations," *Administrative Science Quarterly*, 7 (December 1962), 349–64.

doors are locked in the evening she is as much an inmate as any of the patients. In short, she is a social isolate. It is under this condition, then, that she turns to the bureaucratic rules, which provide her with the necessary legitimate support for her behavior. One of the evening attendants on the ward showed considerable insight into her particular position when, in talking with the observer about hospital rules, she said:

> You have to have some definite rules to work with these patients. If you don't they'll try to run things. The rules back you up. *If you don't have the rules to fall back on, what have you got?*

Thus, although the day attendant would also agree that you "have to have some definite rules to work with these patients," she would proceed to construct her own rules. In doing so, she would feel quite secure, because she has available other sources of support, in the event that she is challenged about running the ward as she sees fit. The evening attendant must fall back on formal rules as the supportive foundation for her behavior.

Another difference in social support between the two shifts concerns their responsibility and liability for their actions. The day attendant is responsible for her actions, but is not necessarily liable for the consequences of these actions. That is, she can, in many ways, involve others in the negative consequences of her actions and thereby gain support from them. An example of this mutual involvement mechanism is contained in the following incident.

Helen S., a patient on Ward X, is going home for a short visit. She and her mother, who has come for her, go to the nurses' office to say goodbye, return to Helen's room to get her belongings together, and then leave the ward without returning to the office. About half an hour later, Mrs. Talbot notices a small bottle containing medication capsules on the counter in front of the medicine cabinet and exclaims, "Oh, my goodness. I forgot to give Helen her medicine to take with her." She spends the next fifteen minutes trying to figure out what she should do—she can't deliver the medication herself, or expect Helen's mother to make another trip because she lives some distance away. Should she notify the doctor and have some arrangement made to get the medication to Helen? In the process of weighing alternatives, Mrs. Talbot voices a number of questions to the observer: "Why didn't Helen remember to pick up her medicine? She's been home before and knows she has to take her medication with her. How was I to know that they weren't coming back to the nurses' office to pick up the medicine?" Mrs. Talbot then makes three phone calls: one to the ward attendant upstairs, a second to the pharmacist who made up Helen's medication order, and a third to the ward physician.

To the upstairs ward attendant, Mrs. Talbot says that Helen went on leave without taking her medication; she indicates that Helen did not return to the nurse's office to pick up the medication that was left there for her.

Of the pharmacist, Mrs. Talbot inquires why the medication had been sent to the ward, and not kept at the pharmacy where it would be picked up by Helen's mother. Mrs. Talbot indicates that this procedure had been used in the past, and asks whether the pharmacist had been directed by the doctor to send the medication over. [According to the formal hospital rule, the pharmacist is not to release a medication order without a written request. This rule is rarely in force concerning patients going home on leave, for the pharmacist will release the medication after a phone call from the ward doctor.] After this, Mrs. Talbot tells the pharmacist that Helen has forgotten to take her medication with her when she left the ward, and points out that these things should be guarded against by requiring the person picking up the patient to get the necessary medication from the pharmacy.

In the final phone call to the ward doctor, Mrs. Talbot again reports that Helen has left the hospital without her medication. Mrs. Talbot asks whether the doctor has talked with Helen's mother, and whether he mentioned to her that Helen still has to take her medicine home. The call ends with the ward doctor indicating that he will see that the medictaion gets to Helen.

This incident reveals the opportunities available to day-shift personnel to gain support for any negative consequences of their actions. Mrs. Talbot can be seen as attempting both to explain away an error and to create a diffuse locus of blame for the consequences of her action or lack of action.

Clearly, the evening attendant has no such opportunities for relocating or distributing the blame for any negative consequences of her actions. She has both the responsibility and the liability for actions, and these may function as constraints upon any possible innovative behavior she might consider. In addition, she is cut off from an interpersonal setting in which she could in some way soften the seriousness of errors, and in which she could build up any significant backlog of unpaid obligations that might help her in a time of trouble.

It should also be noted that any errors made by an evening-shift attendant will come to the attention of the day staff on the ward, when the evening attendant is not there to defend herself. For example, she may forget to log an order. When such an error comes to the attention of the day-shift attendants, it is potentially available also to the eyes and ears of the ward attendant, ward doctor, ward nurse, area supervisor, chief of nursing services, and so on. The same error made by a day attendant and discovered by the evening attendant is not readily available to any of the key staff in the upper hierarchy. None of these staff members is present, and the evening attendant can make the error known to them only by specifically making a point of telling them, which is not too likely.

Thus, the evening attendant's responsibility and liability for her actions constitute an added feature of the social-distance patterns that exist between her and the ward doctor. Both factors tend to discourage the evening attendant from exhibiting innovative behavior, and encourages greater compliance with formal rules. The rules, so to speak, have become the major supportive basis for her actions on the ward.

SOME THERAPEUTIC CONSEQUENCES

What are the consequences of these different patterns of social distance which exist between doctors and attendants on the day versus the evening shift? Are the consequences limited only to matters of compliance with rules and maintenance of authority, or do they have implications for staff behavior toward patients? In particular, is it possible that an attendant's effectiveness as a therapeutic agent is influenced by the nature of the doctor-attendant relationship?

Let us begin to examine these questions by looking at the reactions of day- and evening-shift attendants to the three groups of patients discussed in the previous chapter. It will be remembered from Chapter Four that three groups of patients were differentiated according to the number of sociometric choices which they received from other patients along the dimensions of liking and leadership. One group of well-liked patients was designated as Hi Positives; one group of disliked patients was designated as Hi Negatives; and one group of patients selected for leadership was designated as Hi Leaders.

Day- and evening-shift attendants were asked to express their views on how "well" or "sick" they thought all the patients were on their ward and how "well" or "sick" they thought the patients were in each of the three groups described above. Evening shift attendants assigned higher average "sickness" scores to all the patients in their charge. They also assigned much higher "sickness" evaluations to the Hi Positives, Hi Negatives, and Hi Leaders than did the day-shift attendants. Especially noteworthy about these differences is the fact that the day attendants assigned extremely low "sickness" scores to the Leaders, while the evening attendants gave them the second highest "sickness" scores. In light of the finding that Hi Leaders posed the greatest power threat to attendants (see Chapter Four), the reaction of the evening attendants is consistent with the hypothesis that the greatest sensitivity to patient threats would occur on the evening shift, where attendants have fewer mechanisms to protect themselves against threats.

Additional data consistent with the above hypothesis are found in an examination of the custodial attitudes of day- and evening-shift attendants. Gilbert and Levinson's *Custodial Mental Illness Ideology Scale*[13] is designed to measure the presence of a traditional custodial orientation toward the care and treatment of patients. Evening-shift attendants on Ward X had significantly higher custodialism scores than did attendants from the day shift.

Thus, the evening-shift attendant, who is cut off from opportunities for contact with her peers as well as her superordinates, develops a defensive posture toward patients which we described as a tendency to maximize social distance from them. This tendency is indicated by the evening attendants' expression of a more custodial attitude toward patients as well as a greater inclination to see those in her charge as "less normal" than do day attendants. In each case, the reactions of the evening attendants toward patients are not conducive to the emergence or maintenance of a therapeutic milieu.

[13] Doris C. Gilbert and Daniel J. Levinson, "'Custodialism' and 'Humanism' in Mental Hospital Structure and Staff Ideology," in *The Patient and the Mental Hospital*, Milton Greenblatt, Daniel J. Levinson, and Richard H. Williams, eds. (Glencoe, Ill.: Free Press, 1957), pp. 20–35.

The differences between day- and evening-shift attendants described above are apparently not peculiar to Ward X alone. Data obtained from a questionnaire which was distributed to all hospital staff personnel indicated that in contrast to day attendants, evening-shift attendants throughout the hospital were more custodial in their attitudes toward patients and more rule-oriented in their relationships with them.[14]

This analysis suggests that efforts to improve patient care by (1) building more therapeutic attitudes toward patients, (2) increasing respect for and acceptance of patients as people who have worth and value equal to that of staff, and (3) increasing flexibility in the application of rules can occur only if attendants who have the most contact with patients also feel secure and valued as persons and employees themselves. Unfortunately, change in the feelings and behavior of attendants toward patients will not occur without change in the entire authority structure of the hospital; at present this structure is designed to provide custody of societal rejects.

[14] Carolyn Cummings and Robert Perrucci, "Social Distance and Status Protection in a Psychiatric Hospital," *Sociological Quarterly*, 7 (Autumn 1966), 423–35.

III

BECOMING NORMAL

Heroes and Hopelessness: Patients' Release Ideology and Its Breakdown

If, as we suggested in Chapter Two, mental hospitals exist for the main purpose of providing custody for society's rejects and not for the purpose of returning patients to society, then it must be expected that both patients and staff will find a way to accommodate to that fact. Patients and staff could, of course, develop the view that the hospital is nothing more than a "storehouse," but this is unlikely, for it would be a personally painful belief. More likely, they will develop ideas, beliefs, and "evidence" which either supports the view that the hospital does indeed treat, cure, and release persons or explains why the hospital does not do better in the areas of treatment, cure, and discharge.

In this chapter we will examine the ideas and beliefs held by patients about the possibilities for and the procedures by which patients obtain a discharge. It is a collective view of reality that must be "constructed" and is thereby subject to a "test" as to its accuracy. Thus, we shall examine the way a "release ideology" is constructed and the consequences that follow an unsuccessful "test."

COLLECTIVE DISTURBANCE AND SOCIAL CONTROL

The study of internal disorders and the breakdown of social control in institutional settings has long provided an excellent opportunity for an analysis of the sources of strain and stability in organizations. Studies of this type have been concerned with what has been called a "collective disturbance" or a "riot." These terms have been used to denote the fact that the phenomenon under consideration is not an individual disturbance or an aggregate of individual disturbances, but a disturbance that has a contagious element that is transmitted in an interpersonal context. As Stanton and Schwartz describe it, "the collective disturbance involves the participation of a number of people in such a way that *the disturbance of one patient is integrated with the disturbance of many other patients.*" [1]

In seeking to locate the source of a collective disturbance on a psychiatric ward, Stanton and Schwartz focused primarily upon covert staff disagreements and disruptions of normal communication channels.[2] The consequences of these internal disruptions were seen in the increased disturbances of many patients, the magnifying of staff problems such as errors in technique, distorted messages, increased absenteeism, and the partial withdrawal of staff members from normal participation on the ward.

In another study of a psychiatric hospital, Caudill traced a collective disturbance to strains created by an imbalance between affective and cognitive communication among staff members. This in turn led to staff disagreements that were still, for the most part, covert and unexpressed. That is, the disagreements tended to become part of discussions of plans for individual patients, who then became the vehicles through which the disagreements were expressed. A later stage in the disturbance was characterized by the mutual withdrawal of staff groups, which cut the channels of communication between patients and staff, and within staff groups. The still covert nature of the disagreements led to the formation of various support-seeking coalitions, which Caudill labels as "paired role group responses." [3] The final "restitution" phase, or the return to equilibrium, occurred when the "real" disagreements between staff members were openly discussed.

Looking at prison riots, Bates suggests that one of the direct causes of the tensions which burst forth in riot and disorder is due

[1] Alfred H. Stanton and Morris S. Schwartz, *The Mental Hospital* (New York: Basic Books, 1954), p. 382.

[2] *Ibid.*, Chapter 17.

[3] William Caudill, *The Psychiatric Hospital as a Small Society* (Cambridge, Mass.: Harvard University Press, 1958).

to the enforced idleness of the inmates.[4] His hypothesis suggests that a certain amount of free-floating tension will, from time to time, manifest itself in various types of disturbances.

What we find lacking in these discussions of collective disturbances is any explicit analysis of the disturbances in terms of the state of the system as it operates as a mechanism of social control. For example, the Stanton and Schwartz definition of a collective disturbance could very well include the case of an individually disturbed patient who upsets other patients by her presence and behavior. Thus, the contagion aspect of the disturbance might be only that the other patients get upset by the mere presence of a patient in their midst who is extremely disturbed, hostile, or critical. This possibility is strongly suggested in both the Stanton and Schwartz and the Caudill studies, in that each of them presents the situation of a peculiarly disturbed or obnoxious patient or patients as key figures in the overall collective disturbance.

In this chapter we shall also examine a collective disturbance. However, our concern will be with (1) the patient's conception of what constitutes the release process, or the chain of events in a patient's life that leads to a release from the hospital; (2) the extent to which the patient's release ideology fits the actual release process; and (3) the consequences of maintaining an ideology which does not fit the real situation. These three elements are seen as linked to the general question of social control in the hospital and as specifically involved in the sequence of events leading to a collective disturbance on the ward.

SOME PRECONDITIONS FOR THE DISTURBANCE

A good many of the patients on Ward X have been through the "treatment mill." During their present hospitalization and in previous ones, they have been exposed to one or another of the physical, chemical, mechanical, or analytic therapies available in psychiatric practice. It is by no means unusual to find patients who

[4] Sanford Bates, *A Statement Concerning Causes, Preventive Measures, and Methods of Controlling Prison Riots and Disturbances* (New York: American Prison Association, 1953), p. 10.

have had insulin shock, electroshock, lobotomy, group therapy, individual therapy, drugs, and assorted occupational and recreational therapies. Given the considerable amount of existing treatment that has already been received by most patients, what can one expect of the ward physician who has the responsibility of trying to provide some therapeutic program for these patients? As might be expected, the ward physician, in large part, adopts the pose of the surgeon who has just completed a difficult operation saying, "I've done all I can, it's out of my hands now." The responsibility for getting "well" again somehow winds up in the hands of the patients themselves. As one physician put it, in speaking of Ward X patients: "A lot of them here are somewhere between the hospital and the community, but they won't get off the seat of their pants. If they don't make a move, there's nothing we can do for them." Similarly, the ward physician, in response to the numerous questions such as, "When can I go home?" or "Am I getting any better?" or "Do you think I'm ready to go to staff?" will generally respond, "I can't tell you that, Mary; you've got to tell me when you're ready to go home."

In many respects, then, the patient is thrown back on her own resources to get estimates of just how well she is or isn't doing. Patients thus become overly sensitive to the little nuances of staff behavior which they take to be signs full of important meanings. For example, in an attempt to cheer up a patient who had been very depressed for several days, the ward attendant called her into the office and offered her a relatively new winter coat that a volunteer worker had donated (it was late July at the time). While the patient tried on the coat, the ward nurse and attendant both commented on how well it fitted her and how nice she looked in it. After listening to them for a few moments, the patient turned to them and said, "In other words, I'll be here this winter."

Thus, in this setting, we find a fertile ground for the emergence of various belief systems dealing with the problem of obtaining various indications of one's therapeutic position on the ward. Patients must draw upon their own experiences and resources to come to terms with the most pressing problem facing them—namely, how to get out. What they do not know, however, is that the staff is a full partner in their ignorance about how one knows when it is "time" to be released. In response to this situation, what we find on Ward X is the emergence of what we will call a "release ideology," or a collection of beliefs referring to available means for obtaining a release from the hospital.

THE CONSTRUCTION OF A RELEASE IDEOLOGY

Every social system that persists long enough to develop a history generally creates "culture heroes." These figures, either real or fictitious, are thought to reflect the most highly valued qualities of the culture; and as such they often become, in a vague sort of way, a potential source of culturally approved aspirations for group members. In this respect, the mental hospital also creates its culture heroes. On Ward X in particular, these heroes tend to be patients who have "made it," who have been released from the hospital. Thus, these culture figures may be viewed as reflecting the most highly valued patient aspiration—that of getting out of the hospital.

The creation of culture heroes, however, does not occur only among the patients. Ward staff are quite instrumental in influencing the patients' concern with exemplary heroes. For example, ward attendants are repeatedly telling and retelling the success stories of patients who went from being incontinents on a back ward to rehabilitated members of society. It is a clear counterpart to the Horatio Alger myth, only in a psychiatric setting. The main reason attendants seem to retell these success stories is due primarily to the relative absence of cases in which the attendants can illustrate how they helped patients to recover. Thus, in the success stories, the attendants can indicate the role they themselves played in the rehabilitation process.

With this impetus from ward staff, the attention of the patients themselves also tend to focus upon these success stories. For one thing, the patients probably hope they can enjoy some of the praise which attendants heap upon the heroes for real or alleged behavioral or personality characteristics. For another, it becomes a tangible piece of evidence from which they may judge their own stage of progress in the hospital; a piece of evidence which, as we indicated earlier, is not forthcoming from the ward physician or other hospital staff.

In the actual "putting together" of the ideology, the patients tend to focus upon the most prominent features of the culture heroes' life in the hospital, especially in the period of time just prior to discharge. On Ward X, the prominent features of exemplary heroes that patients seemed to isolate most often were the following:

1. *Working with Companion Service*—this involves a patient-organized and patient-run service to the hospital (with staff supervision) whereby the participating patients provide an escort service to all wards of the hospital. They escort single patients or groups of patients to and from activities, appointments, and the like, thereby releasing considerable time for the regular hospital staff to turn to more important work. This program has received much publicity both within and outside the hospital, and is considered a very desirable position by most patients.

2. *Coming off medication*—as this implies, it simply means a ward physician's decision to take a patient off any mood-elevating or tranquilizing drug program.

3. *Becoming a patient leader*—what we generally find here is the recognition of the formal patient leader, in terms of the elected ward president or vice-president. Thus, the leadership role would exclude informal leaders, because they would not have the recognition and approval of the hospital staff members.

4. *Getting along well with ward staff*—this is the loosest or vaguest characteristic of the culture heroes which the patients recognize. It generally means that a patient "talks well" with staff members; that they engage in extended conversations on topics which transcend the patient-staff role relationships. For example, the freedom to walk into the nurses' office and sit down and chat with the attendants, or more important, to be taken into the confidence of a ward staff member.

These are the four main factors that the patients tend to isolate in reflecting upon the prerelease behavior of the culture heroes. In most cases, these four factors quite accurately characterize the prerelease behavior of discharged patients. We would suggest that the reason these characteristics are manifested by the culture heroes is that they are the *results* or *consequences* of a poorly understood process of "getting better." That is, the patient who is making good progress "putting himself together again" will be very likely to go on Companion Service, to come off medication, to become a patient leader, and to get on well with ward staff. However, in the creation of the release ideology, these four characteristics are viewed as *things to be done in order to get better*. The patients on the ward take the behavioral manifestations of the "getting better" process and make them the *causes* of the process. This reversal of cause and effect has been noted by Schneider and Dornbusch in a very different context; applied to Ward X we would say that the patients have taken certain latent functions of the recovery process and made them manifest by pursuing them as goals.[5] What had previously been realized as a by-product is now instrumentalized as a means for attaining mental health.

THE CONCRETIZATION OF THE IDEOLOGY

The release ideology described above allows the patients to maintain the belief that there is a clear-cut way to get better and get out of the hospital. The actual reality of the belief system is never an issue, because it has been created out of rather reliable evidence (i.e., discharged patients), and also because it has never been shown not to be true. That is, the only patients who have ever embodied these four ideological characteristics have been the culture heroes. Aside from them, several patients may have one or two of the characteristics, such as working on Companion Service and getting on well with ward staff, but never all four characteristics.

In this part of the process of the collective disturbance, we will describe the case of the patient who did embody all four characteristics—the "concretization" of the ideology. This is the case of Marie I.; a patient who represented the unfolding of Ward X's Horatio Alger myth. Marie I. came onto Ward X during the last week in May. She came to the ward with what might be considered "poor credentials." That is, she was not the most desirable type of patient for an open ward. The ward attendant, upon hearing of Marie's transfer, made the following comment. "Well, we're getting two new girls. Dr. Brown said we're getting one good one and one of the other kind. The good one is Sally T., the other girl is

[5] Louis Schneider and Sanford Dornbusch, *Popular Religion* (Chicago: University of Chicago Press, 1959), esp. pp. 58–77.

Marie I. She's coming from a back ward; a real fighter. I don't know how they expect us to help her on this ward."

On the ward two days later, the day attendant pointed out Marie I. to the observer.

"That's Marie. She came over from 14 [*the disturbed ward*]. You'd better watch out for her; when she blows, she really blows. I feel sorry for the night attendant. She can sure have trouble sometimes, especially with girls like Marie."

The first two weeks on the ward for Marie I. were rather uneventful. She was immediately assigned to a job doing housework in another building, which she did without difficulty. Her medication program included several depressants, which she took without incident. Aside from a few minor evening complaints of inability to sleep and several physical complaints requiring absence from work, Marie was a good patient. She was good in the sense of being unobtrusive, keeping to herself, and causing no difficulties for other patients or ward staff.

On June 20, Marie had her first extended contact with the ward physician during office hours. The interview was a pleasant one, with the doctor indicating his interest in Marie's condition and the importance, to Marie, of this move to an open ward. The doctor stressed the fact that this was probably an important turning point in her illness. Marie was clearly pleased with the doctor, and repeatedly stated how much she liked the ward, the staff, and the other patients.

At this point Marie was observed to have become much more outgoing. She established a close friendship with Mary G., one of the very well-liked patients on the ward. The ward staff also became sensitive to the fact that Marie was "coming out of her shell." On June 29, Mrs. Talbot, the day attendant, made the following reply to Dr. Powell's inquiry concerning Marie. "She's getting along real fine. She fits in well, and most of the girls really like her. Just the other morning she went by the office door and said, 'Hi [nickname].' Well, my head just shot up. She came back and apologized because she thought I was mad. Well, I wasn't, it was just a surprise to hear her say that. A lot of the old-timers call me that, but a new girl usually won't."

On July 1, the ward president received a six-month leave of absence. A special election was held, and Marie I. was elected the new president. The ward staff, and by extension, the patients, made quite a bit of "noise" about it. At attendant lunches or coffee breaks, Marie became a living testimonial to the therapeutic atmosphere of Ward X. "A little over a month ago she was fighting and scratching on a back ward, and now she's president of the ward council," was the comment of the day attendant.

On July 12, the evening shift attendant wrote the following unsolicited progress note on Marie:

This patient has shown a wonderful improvement on my time since she first came on this ward. She is no longer a sleeping problem. She sleeps all night. She gets up very bright and cheerful at 5:30 A.M.

During this time, Marie made a definite effort to convince the ward attendants and ward physician that she no longer needed her medication. Each time the ward physician came for office hours, Marie managed to see him and repeat her request. On July 20, the following note appeared in Marie's chart:

Patient asked doctor to have her medication discontinued again. Discontinue Thorazine and Dulcolox. Reduce Equanil to 200 mg.

At this point in Marie's stay on Ward X she had managed to exhibit the four most highly valued factors which made up the release ideology. She was an escort for Companion Service; she was ward president; she was off medication; and she got along very well with ward staff. Regardless of the "workability" of the ideology in actually yielding the desired result of a release from the hospital, a patient who exhibited these four characteristics should carry a rather favorable prognosis. For Marie I., however, we find a very rapid process of deterioration setting in; a transition even more marked than her meteoric rise from a back ward to a ward hero. We will now turn to Marie's individual "breakdown," and the manner in which it affected the other patients on the ward.

THE IDEOLOGY PUT TO THE TEST

The rapid decline of Marie I. made its first appearance with the news that two patients on Ward X were in the planning stage for a release from the hospital. Although plans had apparently been in progress for some time through the Social Service Department, it now became public ward information that Carla W. was being considered for a six-month leave of absence, and Lizzie S. was under consideration for a work placement. Neither of these two patients was very popular on the ward. In fact, Lizzie S. was one of the patients receiving the highest number of negative sociometric choices (a Hi Negative in Chapter 4). In addition, the news of these plans was not met with the wholehearted approval of the ward attendants. As Mrs. Talbot put it:

> I can't understand it. Neither Carla nor Lizzie is ready to leave here; they're both very disturbed. Not that I'm not glad to get rid of them, but they'll never make it. They shouldn't even be considered for leaves.

This news became public on July 26. On July 27, Lizzie S. was put *on* additional medication (Reserpine). On July 28 and 29, the following notes were written in Marie I.'s chart.

> Patient came to office with a thin blouse on and a pair of jeans. Told her to go get a brassiere and slip on because you could see through the blouse. Said she was alright, no one could see through her. Just stood and stared at me. After a while she finally put on a dress. Said she didn't like to be told about her clothes. Patient seems very nervous. First complaining of constipation and was given laxative. This patient stated bowels acted some. Stayed on ward this P.M. saying didn't feel well. Is trying hard to get upset. Is disturbed at times. Is irritable and very unreasonable. Patient came to office saying she might as well go back to work for she had to listen to Celine's radio. Tried to talk with patient but she became very sullen and held her mouth open running her tongue around the inside of her mouth and stared into space. Patient went to room to rest up.

On July 31, the following note was written on Carla W.

> Patient given medication for upset stomach. Patient restless, found her crying. Stated she was having bad dreams. Was very unhappy all evening.

The following three notes were written on Lizzie S. for July 30, 31, and August 1, respectively.

> This patient has been getting up for last week complaining of pains in stomach. States she has a lot of diarrhea.
> Patient has been very talkative several times during night. Very restless.
> Patient put on Equanil to relieve anxiety.

On August 3, the following note was written on Marie I.

Patient is very strong against Elsa P. sleeping next to her. She is continually calling her names to this attendant. States Elsa watches her all the time.

On August 6, both Carla W. and Lizzie S. were released from the hospital on a leave of absence and a work placement, respectively. The departure of these two patients was discussed by the ward attendant and ward nurse in the following manner.

ATTENDANT Well, Carla went out, but was she high. She went around demanding that things be done for her. She said to me, "I demand that you call [social worker] about me going home." I don't know how they let her go. Just two days ago the doctor gave orders to seclude her or send her to [closed ward] if she acted up, and today they let her out.

NURSE Lizzie was just as disturbed. Monday she told me that Beth L. was threatening to kill her, and she started crying. Anyway, I'm glad to see her go.

With the release of these two patients we find a move into the acute stage of the disturbance. For up to this point (July 29 to August 6), what we found was primarily the individual upset of Marie I. The rest of the patients on the ward were apparently affected only to the extent that there appeared to be a marked increase in complaints about physical ailments.[6] Thus, the acute phase of the disturbance involved the "complete breakdown" of Marie I. (by staff definitions, this involves a psychotic episode and the return to a closed ward), as well as a number of extreme upsets of other patients that were presumably related to Marie's disturbance. We will relate each incident by the day of occurrence and the patient involved.

August 7: Marie I., nursing note, day shift.

Patient has burning sensation when she urinates. Patient said she felt stuffy, and needed a bowel movement.

[6] It is interesting to note in this context that the one and only case of bed-wetting on Ward X (during the field study) occurred during the disturbance phase. On August 3 and 4, Joan B. became incontinent. At this time she was "specialed" by the evening and night attendants. That is, she was awakened periodically during the night and taken to the bathroom. She was generally awakened at 11:00 P.M. and 3:00 A.M. This solved the bed-wetting problem, but then Joan became a "problem sleeper"; i.e., it was very difficult getting her up in the morning.

August 8: Marie I., day shift, observations on the ward.

MARIE   Could I have a soda mint or bicarb?

NURSE   Why?

MARIE   So I can belch.

NURSE   Are you under tension at work, Marie?

MARIE   [*laughs*] Who isn't under tension here? Can I have a soda mint?

NURSE   Well, Marie, you know what we are trying to do here is to get you people off medications. You can't always be running for a soda mint or a bicarb when you get out.

MARIE   Well, I'm sure I can get a bicarb if I need it.

(*Marie walked away from the office into the day room and out to the loggia. She spoke of the incident to a group of patients who were smoking in the loggia*)

MARIE   She told me, "we don't want you to get used to the medication" [*in a mimicking voice*]. I'll get my own stuff to burp. I can spend a dime on a coca cola so she won't have to chart a soda mint. They don't worry about shock treatments becoming habit-forming, but they worry about soda mints.

August 9: Marie I., nursing note, evening shift.

Patient very disturbed. Was restless and fault-finding all evening. Attendant talked with her at 7:00 P.M. She quieted down for a while. Later came in office while supervisor was here. She walked up to medicine cabinet and tried to open it. She was very angry to find it locked. Threatened the supervisor. Attendant talked with her again. She threatened her life; also stated she would run away if doctor did not transfer her to Ward _____. Was very insulting to some of the other patients. Seemed to think she was as well or even better than two of the patients that had been sent out on work placement. Patient was watched very close.

August 10: Marie I., day shift, observations on the ward.

Marie went to work on Companion Service at 8:30 A.M. At 10:15 A.M. Marie was brought back to the ward by the attendant in charge of the service. The patient was very upset and crying. Mrs. Talbot, the ward attendant, asked Marie what was the matter. Marie stated, "If we'd get rid of Beth L. and Betty L. [*two other patients on the ward*], things would go a lot better on this ward."

(MRS. TALBOT *helped* MARIE *to her room to lie down.* DR. POWELL *was called and he came right over. Marie was asked to come to the nurses' office and talk with him.*)

DR. POWELL I understand you've been a little upset, Marie. You want to tell me about it?

MARIE It's this whole goddamn place. You ask for a soda mint and they make a big deal out of it. I tried to get some powder from the medicine cabinet and the attendant and the supervisor jumped on me. They told me that the office was for the nurses and attendants and that I should stay out.

DR. POWELL You have to understand that there are some rules round here, Marie. Don't you think you have to abide by the rules?

MARIE Yes, I know there are rules, I've been following them for weeks. I was the good Marie, the sweet Marie. I worked hard to go on Companion Service and to get along without my medicine, and what did it get me? [*Patient starts crying at this point.*] You let Carla and Lizzie go out, and I was better than either of them. Lizzie even went on medicine before she went out.

DR. POWELL Well, what do you want me to do, Marie? You think I should let you go home?

MARIE I want to go to Ward [*closed ward*]. At least over there I can cry and no one looks at you as if something's wrong.

DR. POWELL I'll tell you what. Why don't you go lie down and rest and we can talk again later.

MARIE I don't give a shit for your medicine or your hospital.

(MARIE *gets up and walks out of the office.* MRS. TALBOT *goes after her and gets her to lie down in her room.* MRS. TALBOT *returns to the office.*)

MRS. TALBOT You think we should send her over to [*closed ward*]? She's going to blow any minute.

DR. POWELL Let's hold her here for now. She's made such great strides these past months, I'd hate to set her back without a good try. Keep her in her room and keep an eye on her once in a while. I'll talk to her tomorrow.

That noon at lunchtime, Marie did not go to lunch with the ward but remained in her room. The Ward X attendant escorted the patients from Wards X and Y to the dining room. The attendant from Ward Y (upstairs) was to keep an eye on the Ward X patients who do not go to regular lunch. When the Ward X attendant and the observer returned to the ward, the following incident was reported by the Ward Y attendant.

I was upstairs in the office when all of a sudden I heard a big racket coming from below. There was some yelling and screaming. I ran downstairs and there at the end of the hall were Marie I. and Beth L. rolling around and fighting on the floor. It was a job getting them apart, but I finally got them in their own rooms. I couldn't get anything out of Marie because she's been crying all this time. Beth told me that she was in her room minding her own business when Marie walked in and called her a "goddamn whore" and started hitting her and pulling her hair. Marie picked on the wrong one this time, because Beth was really giving it to her when I got down here.

Mrs. Talbot called Dr. Powell and reported the incident. Marie was immediately sent over to a closed ward. Later that evening, and through the night, a number of additional incidents occurred. However, it becomes most difficult to establish anything like a causal link between Marie I.'s disturbance and the subsequent upsets of several other patients. At this point, we will only relate the incidents and then attempt to establish their relationship to Marie's disturbance. Reported below is the statement made by the day attendant to the observer on August 11, the day after Marie I. was sent to a closed ward.

Last night it was really a madhouse here. You knew that Marie "blew" yesterday, didn't you? Well, that's not the all of it. About 8:00 last night, Mary G. went psychotic. She was running up and down the hall yelling and singing hymns. Then she started talking to God, saying how sorry she was and all that. Minton [*evening attendant*] said it was a real mess. They sent her over with Marie I. on [*closed ward*]. Then to top it all off, Elizabeth K. tried to choke Julia T. in the middle of the night. Julia started yelling and practically woke up the whole ward. They moved Elizabeth to the empty room at the end of the hall, and they're going to keep her door locked at night.

Aside from these remarks by the day attendant, the observer also noted some additional incidents which may or may not have been relevant to the disturbance. However, their occurrence at this particular time—i.e., at the acute stage of the disturbance—makes them potentially relevant. The incidents simply involve three patients who did not go to work on August 11. Wanda R., Bertha G., and Betty L. all claimed that they were not feeling good, for one reason or another, and wished to be excused from work.

As we stated above, the causal connection between Marie I.'s disturbance and the subsequent upsets of other patients is difficult to establish. The one common element in all these events is their occurrence in a certain time sequence. Aside from this, it would be difficult to explain the connections among *all* these events. Nevertheless, the following explanation is offered.

The "psychotic episode" of Mary G., which followed very closely the disturbance of Marie I., is most interesting in view of the fact that Mary G. and Marie I. were very close friends on the ward. On the sociometric questionnaire, they were among the few pairs of mutual friendship choices made by patients. Thus, there does seem to be some likelihood that the two disturbances were connected. The other significant feature of all of the disturbances that followed Marie I.'s is the fact that they occurred among relatively active patients holding significant status positions within the patient group. For example, of the six patients involved in these upsets, five were patients who were either very popular or very unpopular according to our sociometric questionnaire. Mary G., Elizabeth K., and Wanda R. were all among the patients most frequently chosen for potential roommates (Hi Positives in Chapter 4); Julia T. was one of the two ward leaders (Hi Leaders in Chapter 4); and Betty L. was one of the most frequently negatively selected patients (Hi Negatives in Chapter 4). Thus, it is quite possible that, because they were all active patients, they were perhaps more sensitive to the symbolic meaning of the breakdown of Marie I.: that is, that her disturbance represented a breakdown of the release ideology. It is with respect to the release ideology that we would expect the active patients to be concerned, because they would be more likely to be cognizant of the presumed utility of the ideology in attaining a release from the hospital.

UNATTAINABLE GOALS AND THE COLLECTIVE DISTURBANCE

In the preceding section, a description of the events leading to a collective disturbance on the ward was outlined in some detail. The actual disturbance itself was seen as intimately connected to the release ideology; an ideology which provided a framework of instrumental means for the attainment of a certain goal. As we have tried to indicate, the ideology was badly constructed. That is, the specific means isolated by the patients bore no relationship to the indicators used by staff to establish a patient's release prognosis if, in fact, the staff have such indicators (see the next chapter for a discussion of this point). Thus, in the last analysis, behavior in accordance with the ideological prescription did not produce the anticipated results. Aside from this, however, the existence of these strong beliefs about the release process raises some further questions concerning the persistence of "magic" within the rationalized framework of the hospital. We had earlier characterized the Ward X patients as persons who are on their own in the construction of a belief system that makes their institutional life bearable. We might also add to this the fact that Ward X patients are attempting to do this without really workable knowledge and are therefore receptive to "magical" practices.

Thus, we might posit the functional necessity, for the maintenance of order in the hospital, of a belief system which attests to the existence of "real" treatment procedures, treatment effectiveness and, in short, a belief that there is a way to get out of the hospital. However, the "rational" world of the staff very rarely intrudes upon the patient world in the form of providing clear-cut information. For the most part, patients are kept in the dark as to expectations regarding treatment effectiveness and release prognosis, because the staff are also in the dark. The patients, therefore, build an explanatory system which provides this information, and which allows them to accept the normative constraints imposed upon them, as well as legitimizing the authority of those in the hierarchy who exercise control over them. The following statement by Parsons, in discussing some of Malinowski's work on magic, is very relevant for our discussion of the release ideology.

Malinowski, however, went beyond this in attempting to understand the functional necessity for such mechanisms as magic. In this connection, he laid stress on the importance of the emotional interests involved in the successful outcome of such enterprises. *The combination of a strong emotional interest with important factors of uncertainty, which on the given technical level are inherent in the situation, produces a state of tension and exposes the actor to frustration.* This, it should be noted, exists not only in cases where uncontrollable factors, such as bad weather or insect pests in gardening result in "undeserved" failure, *but also in cases where success is out of proportion to reasonable expectations of the results of intelligence and effort.* Unless there were mechanisms which had the psychological function of mitigating the sense of frustration, the consequences would be unfavorable to maintaining a high level of confidence or effort, and it is in this connection that magic may be seen to perform important positive functions. . . . It would follow that wherever such uncertainty elements enter into the pursuit of emotionally important goals, if not magic, at least functionally equivalent phenomena could be expected to appear.[7]

Thus, while both Parsons and Malinowski point out the functional significance of magic in coping with uncertainty, it is quite clear that the magical beliefs *coexist* with the rational knowledge rather than seeking to *replace* the rational knowledge in a system of goal-directed activity. As Parsons points out:

> Side by side with the system of rational knowledge and technique, however, and specifically not confused with it, was a system of magical beliefs and practices. . . . Correspondingly, the practices were not rational techniques but rituals involving specific orientation to this world of supernatural forces and entities.[8]

It appears in this interpretation that the contribution—i.e., functional significance—the magical system makes to maintaining what we might call some semblance of order in the system comes primarily from the fact that the belief system stands *outside* any expectation of results in goal-directed behavior. In the absence of specific means by which "cures" can be effected and discharges obtained, both patients and staff are forced to construct belief systems that make their respective lives tolerable. The other alternative would be to accept the hospital for what it is: a storehouse of human rejects presided over by caretakers whose only job is to keep them there.

A FINAL NOTE ON MEANS, ENDS, AND ANOMIE

Our use, in this chapter, of notions dealing with the consequences of behavior directed toward unattainable goals, is closely tied to a continued sociological concern with the concept of anomie. In this section, the full theoretical significance of our observations

[7] Talcott Parsons, "The Theoretical Development of the Sociology of Religion," in *Essays in Sociological Theory* (Glencoe, Ill.: The Free Press, 1949), pp. 203–204, emphasis added. It should also be noted that in a footnote to this quoted statement, Parsons also mentions the particular importance of these ideas on magic in the field of health and medicine.

[8] Ibid., p. 202.

on unattainable goals and the collective disturbance will be explored. Specifically, an aspect of Durkheim's concept of anomie will be examined in light of some of our earlier observations.

When the normative system of a society no longer influences and directs the behavior of its members we may say that there is an absence of social control. Individual behavior is no longer a response to collective definitions of the "appropriate," but is, rather, a case of individual determination of behavior. Perhaps the most important study dealing with the breakdown of normative control is Durkheim's *Suicide*.[9] Durkheim was primarily concerned with analyzing the situation in which the means and ends of individual behavior no longer correspond to the normative definitions of means and ends. When the ends of individual action are no longer subject to normative definitions—that is, when a state of *deregulation* of behavior exists—society is said to be characterized by a state or condition of anomie.[10]

Durkheim identified two general conditions in the means-ends system of behavior that give rise to a state of deregulation. The first refers to a condition in which, because of acute changes in society—e.g., economic crises—the means and ends of a system of action that existed *prior* to the crises no longer work. That is, the connection or link between the means-ends action system are inappropriate in a new social context; behavior that once "paid off"—i.e., yielded a desirable end state—is no longer applicable to the new situation. With economic crises, both booms and depressions, Durkheim suggests that "something like a declassification occurs." [11] In describing this he states:

Then, truly, as the conditions of life are changed, the standard according to which most needs are regulated can no longer remain the same. . . . The scale is upset; but a new scale cannot be immediately improvised. Time is required for the public conscience to reclassify men and things. So long as the social forces thus freed have not regained equilibrium, their respective values are unknown and so all regulation is lacking for a time. The limits are unknown between the possible and the impossible, what is

[9] Emile Durkheim, *Suicide*, ed. George Simpson (Glencoe, Ill.: The Free Press, 1951).

[10] Ibid., pp. 246–54.

[11] Ibid., pp. 252.

just and what is unjust, legitimate claims and the hopes of those which are immoderate. Consequently, there is no restraint upon aspirations.[12]

The second condition discussed by Durkheim refers only to the ends or goals of action. Here we find a description of goals that can never be attained; a condition of unattainability of goals because the goals are by definition unattainable.[13] Thus, it is not a case where the means and ends of action are out of joint and must be readjusted, it is a case where the goals could not be attained by any goal-directed means.

Durkheim's analysis of anomie received its fullest elaboration in the now well-known essay by Merton entitled, "Social Structure and Anomie." [14] In addressing himself to the social and cultural sources of deviant behavior, Merton has focused upon the first condition of anomie raised by Durkheim: when the means and ends of action are distributed in society in such a way as to make certain sought-after ends unattainable. As Merton states,

Anomie . . . is a breakdown in the cultural structure, occurring particularly when there is an acute disjunction between the cultural norms and goals and the socially structured capacities of members of the group to act in accord with them. In this conception, cultural values may help to produce the behavior which is at odds with the mandates of the values themselves.[15]

Thus, the emphasis by Merton is on the pressure for deviant behavior which is the result of the selection of normatively proscribed means for the attainment of cultural goals. The outcome of anomie results in a disruption of the normative system in its effectiveness in ensuring conforming behavior. However, it should be noted that the pressures for deviant behavior produces the deviant adaptations primarily within the lower classes. Thus, it is possible that the existence of deviant adaptations may, in fact, *reinforce* the legitimacy of the normative system for the larger society precisely because compliance with *prescribed* means does

12 Ibid., pp. 252–53.

13 Ibid., p. 248.

14 Robert K. Merton, *Social Theory and Social Structure* (Glencoe, Ill.: The Free Press, 1959).

15 Ibid., p. 162.

result in the attainment of desired goals. Put differently, we are suggesting that the existence of deviant adaptations which are the result of the way the system is organized does not necessarily question the legitimacy or moral fiber of the system. Clearly, the deviant has not utilized the appropriate means for attaining his ends, and as long as the system can demonstrate that appropriate means are available and *do work*, the action of the deviant can only deserve the moral disapproval of the society. For example, even though a society may recognize that its lower strata are economically discouraged from attaining higher education, in terms of relative probabilities, there is a sufficient masking overlay from the open class ideology to draw upon examples of the rags-to-riches success story.[16]

The question we are raising here, in a roundabout way, is under what conditions is the legitimacy of the normative system questioned? When will the actors in the system no longer comply with the normative definitions of acceptable means and ends governing behavior? This involves a broader type of normative disruption than concerns Merton. We are thinking here of the kind of moral sickness or *malaise* as described by Durkheim. Individual reactions to such a condition are best described by terms like "demoralization" or "disenchantment." Under such conditions, the legitimacy of norms is discredited, and the usefulness of the existing institutionalized system is questioned.[17]

[16] It is also possible that those who follow the deviant adaptation are also unable to blame the system for their difficulties. Because they have probably been exposed, to some extent, to the examples of "those who have made it" via appropriate means, they would probably turn to a type of self-blame of the "if I had my life to live over again" variety.

[17] It should be noted that the discussion here is very close to Merton's "rebellion" mode of adaptation. He states: "When the institutional system is regarded as a barrier to the satisfaction of legitimized goals, the stage is set for rebellion as an adaptive response" (*Social Theory and Social Structure,* p. 156). The precise question we are asking is: When is the institutional system regarded as a barrier? We suggested earlier that under Merton's means-ends paradigm the legitimacy of the existing system need not be questioned. Merton implies that the prerequisite for rebellion is a stage of "awareness" or "consciousness" of the faults of the system. In this sense, then, our question resembles the Marxian concern of looking for the specific social conditions which are necessary for the proletariat to see the "causal nexus" of the reasons for their class situation.

We suggest that the system will be blamed, so to speak, for failures to attain cultural goals primarily under conditions in which *prescribed and culturally appropriate means have been utilized and the expected ends are still not forthcoming*. It is under these conditions that the normative system is put to the test and found to be lacking, while in the Merton paradigm, the moral fiber of the normative system is not *necessarily* shaken. Here is where we see the second condition of anomie discussed by Durkheim; namely, where the goals are unattainable because of their *nature*, and irrespective of the means of attainment utilized. However, we are primarily concerned here with the situation in which the means used and the goal pursued are *both* culturally approved, yet do not work when they become part of an individual's behavioral system.

The mental hospital is just such a setting where the means and ends of human action seem out of joint, and where myths and collective beliefs exist in order to maintain a collective fiction: that treatment and discharge are the central goals of the hospital. This fiction, as we have pointed out earlier, is necessary to allow the society to deal with the fact that it rejects some of its members; it is necessary for hospital staff in order to maintain their favorable self-concepts; and, as we have shown in this chapter, it is even necessary for the patients in order to avoid accepting the harsh reality of a lifetime in the hospital.

The psychiatric setting seems to generate pressure for converting magical beliefs into rational, technical means designed to achieve specified ends. On the other hand, perhaps the release ideology, which we have called a magical belief (because it is technically unrelated to achieving a release from the hospital), could be viewed as containing reasonable intermediate goals which patients could pursue in their own right and which may result in satisfaction and improvements in institutional life.[18] As intermediate goals, which are readily attainable by patients, they could also be viewed by staff as signs of progress. The difficulty, of course, is that the staff cannot participate in constructing clues, signs, or indicators of

[18] For a discussion of such mechanisms as "gain by indirection" and "attractiveness of intermediates," see Louis Schneider, "The Role of the Category of Ignorance in Sociological Theory: An Exploratory Statement," *American Sociological Review*, 27 (August 1962), 492–508.

progress because they have little control over the actual release process. If they had the power to determine who would and would not be released, and could further require families to accept their former members from the hospital, then they would undoubtedly construct an elaborate system for "measuring" who is ready for discharge. The system so constructed could, of course, be as much a myth as the release ideology, but the power to release would convert a myth into science in short order.

In this chapter we examined how patients dealt with their concerns about getting out of the hospital. In the next chapter we will see how the staff deals with the same concerns.

Going to Staff:
A Search for Release Criteria

The operation of a mental hospital as a system of coordinated activity depends upon its effectiveness in four areas. The hospital must (1) develop a set of standards to determine who shall enter the hospital and who shall not (as we pointed out earlier, these standards are influenced more by agencies external to the hospital); (2) maintain a program of treatment designed to aid a patient toward recovery; (3) provide for patient needs in accordance with a certain level of living; and (4) develop a set of standards to determine who shall leave the hospital and who shall remain. Theoretically, these four areas are interrelated, in that one area develops out of the preceding area, and weaknesses in one area affect all other areas. These four areas strongly suggest the analogy of an industrial organization, where a certain raw material must be transformed into a marketable product. In fact the fourth area—standards regarding release from the hospital—is quite similar to the industrial function of "quality control"; that is, the screening of defective products from reaching the public.

However, the problem of quality control in the mental hospital is not a simple one. The fund of knowledge available for making specific decisions concerning discharge is relatively scarce and elusive, and the power to discharge is not entirely in the hands of those with information and knowledge. For example, in the industrial setting, standards for evaluating the organization's product are rather clear and precise. This is undoubtedly because of the intimate link between the processes utilized to transform a raw material into a finished product, and the standards used to check the quality of the finished product. Similarly, in the prison the problem of quality control is less difficult because the raw material does not have to be transformed in order to be released, but must merely remain a full-time member of the organization. The main criterion is relatively objective, in that the passage of time remains the invariant standard for release.[1] The mental hospital, on the other hand, is not fortunate enough to have clearly objective standards for evaluating its product. Even the actual behavior of the patient, the most objective of the possible standards, cannot be held separate from the different subjective evaluations that can be made of the same behavior.

Thus, we are confronted with the problem of standards for quality control in the mental hospital. How does the hospital judge the relative "wellness" of a patient seeking a release? Are the standards used relevant to the patient in the hospital setting, or in the larger society as well? That is, is the patient who "gets on" well according to hospital standards the patient who will "fall apart" in the outside world? or is the patient who develops a bit of an "institutional neurosis" the one who "makes it" in the larger society? These are clearly very important questions with which the persons involved with denying or granting leaves or discharges must be concerned. Whether precise and specific knowledge is or is not available for making these decisions, certain ground rules must be established to allow hospital staff to operate in this context. We shall be concerned with these ground rules; i.e., the question of standards in quality control. Specifically, we will describe the functions of disposition staff, and the process and meaning of "going to staff." In addition, we will discuss the problem of legitimation in the decision-making process, and examine a number of cases which reveal the various ways in which the actions taken by disposition staff become legitimized.

---

[1] Other criteria for release from the prison are not so objective. The system of merits and demerits certainly affects the amount of time spent in the prison, and such a system is bound to the context of interpersonal relations between inmates and staff. Nonetheless, there is a fixed maximum limit to the time one is required to remain in the system, which gives a greater predictability for release to the prison inmate.

DISPOSITION STAFF

Disposition staff is composed of all physicians having ward responsibilities within a particular treatment service in the hospital. At the time of this study, there were six physicians, including the director of disposition staff, who were generally in attendance at the weekly meetings. In addition, staff is attended by a psychologist, a social worker, and on occasion, an interested nurse or hospital priest or minister. Although there may be participation from the nonmedical staff, it is the medical staff that participates in the final decision-making process.

The function of disposition staff with which we are concerned is its responsibility in granting or denying patient requests for leaves of absence, convalescent leaves, work placements, and discharges.[2] The first three of these requests will be considered as "leaves" while the last will be called "discharges." Each of these two occasions for going to staff differs with respect to who requests the leave or discharge. For example, the idea of seeking a leave generally comes from three possible sources: the patient, the social worker, or the family.[3] However, no matter who initiates the idea concerning a leave, the formal request almost always comes from the family. If a patient initiates the idea, she will write to her family (or tell them during a visit) and ask them to write the doctor requesting a leave of some specified type and duration. If a social worker initiates

[2] The functions of disposition staff are actually much broader. They also concern themselves with decisions regarding a patient's commitment status; for example, whether or not a patient will be granted an extension of a temporary commitment, or whether or not he will be transferred to a regular commitment. In addition, disposition staff is available "for any purpose for which the ward physician may seek consultation." For the purposes of this paper, however, we will only be concerned with disposition staff functions regarding release from the hospital.

[3] What we are here calling the family includes friends, legal guardians, and what the staff likes to call "adoptions"; e.g., a volunteer worker who comes to the hospital once a week may become particularly attached to a patient and begin to take the role of a substitute family. The use of the word "adoption" is also interesting in terms of the many overlapping elements between the "patient role" and the "child role."

the idea, she will also write the family and ask them to request a leave for the patient in question. Thus, the formal request is used primarily to indicate that the family does want the patient home, and are interested in caring for the patient at home.

With a discharge request, we find that staffing proceedings are generally initiated by the patient or ward doctor, and only on occasion by the ward nurse (attendants also initiate the idea by "planting it" with the doctor, but they do not openly pursue the staffing of a patient for discharge). A patient who is continually "on the doctor's back" in expressing a readiness for staff will eventually be met with the doctor's exasperated comment: "All right, if you want to go to staff, we'll send you to staff. Then you can see for yourself if you're ready to leave the hospital." In this situation, the patient will go to staff requesting a discharge without the support of her ward physician.

Once a patient has been scheduled for staffing, the preparation phase begins. This preparation involves the patient's attempt to present her best "self" to staff. Thus, a beauty shop appointment is made for a haircut and/or permanent; facial complexions are religiously worked on by the patient in order to present a clean, well-scrubbed look; a best dress is fixed and cleaned, or if the patient doesn't have a good dress, arrangements are made to borrow one. More important is the preparation made to answer certain expected questions that staff members will ask. Most patients know of approximately a dozen questions that every patient going before staff is asked. This can be seen by looking at the marked similarity of the following six answers given by patients interviewed by the observer, in response to the question: "Can you tell me what kinds of questions patients are asked at staff?"

A. They ask you your name, your age, why you're here. If you think this place has helped you. If you're insane. If you think you should be let out. If they release you, will you do the same things.

A. They asked me if I thought I was better, and if shock treatments helped me out.

A. They delve into your personal business and life too much. They want to find out how you got sick. You have to watch out for arithmetic questions, like subtracting sevens starting from one hundred.

A. The head of staff asks most of the questions. He asks other members if they have anything to ask. He wanted to know if I heard voices, and he asked questions to see if I was in contact with reality, like what time is it? What's the date? Who's the president?

A. Well, they ask about your illness and your condition when you came in. They question you about current events, what your plans are when you leave. You can always depend on being asked if you think the place has helped you. The attendants will usually give you the answers before you go to staff anyway.

A. They usually ask a variety of questions, like how long you were here, why you came, your age, what medication you're on, how much; what it does for you. They generally ask if you feel you've been helped in the hospital. If you've been a problem in the hospital, they'll ask you why, or the circumstances of the problem.

The similarity of these responses is quite an accurate reflection of what actually takes place at staff. An examination of patient folders containing written accounts of staff indicates that the same questions were asked of patients going before staff as long as twenty years ago. The existence of such longstanding traditional elements in the hospital can be seen in a number of other aspects of hospital life. For example, intake interviews, formats for progress notes and nursing notes, and psychological "workups" have remained essentially the same for a good many years.[4]

As one of the above responses also indicated, patients going for staff are "prepped" by ward attendants.[5] They are cautioned to be polite, not to get nervous or excited, and not to criticize anyone on the staff. One of the more interesting pieces of advice given to patients preparing for staff is not to talk too much, but to answer each question as briefly as possible. Thus, patients are instructed to limit the amount (as well as the kind) of information they inject into the staff situation. In a sense, what this piece of advice suggests is that the more you talk, the more likely you are to say something wrong. However the attendants may view this piece of ad-

[4] This aspect of the state mental hospital has also been pointed out in H. Warren Dunham and S. Kirson Weinberg, *The Culture of the State Mental Hospital* (Detroit: Wayne State University Press, 1960).

[5] The attendant's interest in insuring a "good performance" on the part of the patient should be seen in the context of certain superordinate-subordinate relationships which are accompanied by an "education" function. For example, in the teacher-student or parent-child relationship (as well as the attendant-patient relationship), the behavior of the subordinate can always be interpreted as a reflection on the training effectiveness of the superordinate.

vice, we shall try to show later the importance of this aspect of limited information.

Staffing takes place in a rectangular-shaped room approximately 20 feet wide by 40 feet long. At the head of the room behind a large plain desk sits the director of staff. Along one side of the desk is a straight-back chair for the patient; on the other side, a movable blackboard. On the desk are several stacks of master record folders for each patient scheduled to appear before staff that day. The remainder of the room is filled with rows of chairs split by an aisle down the center of the room. Staff physicians and the staff psychologist sit in the rows closest to the front of the room, while social workers, nurses, and clergy sit behind them. Regular attenders at staff can be found to occupy the same seats week in and week out. Outside in the hall the patients waiting to go to staff are accompanied by one or two attendants. There is generally very little conversation among the patients or between the patients and attendants. Because all the patients on the staff list for that day assemble at 1:00 P.M., some will have to wait outside for as long as two or three hours before going in. After being staffed, the patient returns to his or her ward and awaits information from the ward doctor concerning staff's decision.

We will now present a description of staff proceedings in three cases of leave requests that were granted.

CASE 511

DR. HAND   The next one is _____.

DR. STONE   Oh, she'll be here. She's a live one, "hellzapoppin" with her.

(DR. HAND reads briefly from patient's folder, indicating age, sex, race, date of admission, diagnosis, previous hospitalizations, previous leaves, current treatment program. The progress note written by the ward attendant especially for staff is read also. This note usually indicates patient's relationships with others in the ward, and her general cooperativeness or noncooperativeness with ward staff. DR. STONE recommends a leave of absence.)

DR. HAND   Will you call her in, Dr. Craig, and question her? I have to step out for a minute.

(Patient enters and sits down.)

DR. CRAIG:

Q. How long have you been here?
A. About two years.
Q. Have you got a family?
A. No.
Q. You sure you won't have any kids now if you leave?
A. No, I had one of those operations.
Q. Are you going to be an out-patient here?
A. I don't know.

(DR. HAND *returns at this point, and* DR. CRAIG *turns patient over to him.*)

DR. HAND:

Q. Have you ever been on an open ward?
A. No.
Q. You taking any medicine now?
A. Yes.
Q. What are your official plans?
A. I want to go home to my husband.
Q. Are you anxious to go home?
A. Yes.
Q. Does anything bother you?
A. No.
Q. Do you think you need to be here?
A. That's for the doctors to decide.
Q. What happens when you have your nervous breakdowns?
A. I just get all upset, and sometimes I hear voices.
Q. How's the world treating you?
A. O.K.

DR. HAND   Do you want to ask questions, Dr. Miller?

DR. MILLER:

Q. Is your husband working?
A. No, he gets social security checks.
Q. How much does he get?
A. I don't know.

(DR. MILLER *indicates he is done.*)

DR. KIRK *(staff psychologist):*

Q. You say you heard voices—tell us about them.
A. Oh, most of the time they're not too clear.

DR. HAND   When did you hear them last?

PATIENT   Couple of months ago.

DR. KIRK:

Q.   Do the voices make you angry?

A.   No.

Q.   Are there any other signs of mental illness that you have?

A.   Sometimes I think my periods may be some of it. I bleed an awful lot, and just feel terrible that time.

Q.   Do people talk about you?

A.   No.

DR. HAND   Dr. Stone, you want to ask anything?

DR. STONE   No, that's all right.

DR. HAND   O.K., you can leave now, Mrs. _____. Thank you for coming. [PATIENT *leaves.*]

DR. HAND   She takes Thorazine now, 150.

DR. CRAIG   [*to* DR. STONE] Do you think she needs 150?

DR. STONE   She just cooled down. She was high as a kite before.

DR. KIRK   Do you think there's anything significant about her comments on menstrual flow and her illness? Freud said something about it . . .

DR. STONE   [*cutting off* DR. KIRK] Sure he did. I'll give you a lecture on Freud; he was as crazy as a bedbug.

DR. HAND   What shall we do?

DR. STONE   Can't we get Social Service to check on the home before giving her an L.A.? They want her, but I didn't think the home situation was so good.

DR. CRAIG   Let her go home before she gets sicker. She's all right now.

DR. HAND   Let's put her on three months' L.A. instead of six months. That all right with everyone?

(*Everyone gives general support to the director's suggestion.*)

CASE 371

DR. HAND   Let's take _____ next. Dr. Powell has to leave early, so we'll get her now. What about this girl, Dr. Powell?

DR. POWELL   Mr. Holmes [*social worker*] knows this case.

MR. HOLMES   Well, _____ has been here quite a while. She was out on work placement before, and got along pretty well. Now her sister wants her home.

DR. HAND   Have you got the letter requesting her by her sister?

MR. HOLMES   Yes.

DR. HAND   O.K. Bring her in.

(PATIENT *enters and sits down.*)

DR. HAND   Dr. Powell is going to talk to you, Miss _____.

DR. POWELL:

Q. How long have you been in this institution, [*first name*]?

A. I don't know exactly; it's been a good while.

Q. Yes it has; it's been 18 years. You've had lots of visits home, but never stayed home.

(*No response from* PATIENT.)

Q. What brought you here in the first place?

A. I don't know.

Q. You mean you never have figured out why you're in the hospital?

A. No, I've been here so long.

Q. Did you like your work the last time you were out?

A. Yes.

Q. What caused you to come back?

A. I had a lot of arguments with my sister.

Q. What were you arguing about with your sister?

A. It was always over my medicine. She was always taking me to Dr. [*family doctor*] for medicine.

Q. Will you go see Dr. _____ when you're home this time?

A. Yes. But this time I'm going to work. I'm not going to stay home all the time.

Q. Do you think it's best for you to work?

A. Yes.

Q. How much will you get paid?

A. Oh, I don't know.

Q. What kind of work will you do?

A. Office work.[6]

Q. How's your spelling and typing and shorthand?

A. I'll have to brush up on them.

(DR. POWELL *indicates he is finished.*)

DR. HAND   Dr. Miller.

DR. MILLER   Do you prefer office work to housework?

[6] Note in this context that most patients who are making plans to leave the hospital almost invariably indicate their desire for a clerical type of position. This is true in spite of the fact that the great bulk of these patients are from lower-income, lower educational levels. Those patients who have worked prior to or in between hospitalizations have generally held unskilled labor positions; e.g., dishwasher, domestic. This focus on white-collar employment is probably a good reflection of the "middle-classizing" function of hospital resocialization.

PATIENT   Yes.

(DR. MILLER *indicates "that's all."*)

DR. HAND   Question, Dr. Stone?

DR. STONE   No questions.

DR. HAND:

Q.   What have you been doing at the hospital?

A.   I'm a ward worker.

Q.   Will you get along with your sister this time?

A.   Yes, I think so.

Q.   Do you have any other sisters?

A.   No.

Q.   What have we done for you in 18 years?

A.   You've done me lots of good.

Q.   Have voices been bothering you?

A.   No.

Q.   How about dreams?

A.   No.

Q.   Will you take your medicine if you leave?

A.   Yes.

(DR. HAND *nods to* MR. HOLMES.)

MR. HOLMES   You know [*first name*], your sister insists that you cooperate with her this time, if you go to her.

PATIENT   Oh, I will.

DR. HAND   O.K., Miss _____. Thanks for coming.

(PATIENT *exits.*)

DR. HAND   What do you think, Dr. Powell?

DR. POWELL   I think she functions pretty well on the ward.

DR. HAND   The only thing is that she's been here so long.

(*There is a short silence while* DR. HAND *leafs through the patient's folder.*)

(DR. HAND   Well, six months, O.K.

DR. POWELL   I don't think she'll last the six months, personally.

DR. HAND   I agree. She'll be back. Six months then; any other comments?

CASE 471

DR. HAND   Let's take _____ next. She's up for an L.A., and we have to see what to do with her.

DR. POWELL   I think there's a family feud going on there. One person wants her and the other doesn't.

DR. HAND   Is she pretty institutionalized?

DR. POWELL   Yes, she is. I think she'll be all right if someone will take her.

(DR. HAND   *Reads standard information from patient's folder.*)

DR. POWELL   Isn't there a note there from the social worker about the home situation?

(*He goes up and looks through folder and finds no note.*)

DR. HAND   Let's bring her in. Will you start the questioning, Dr. Powell?

(PATIENT *enters.*)

DR. POWELL:

Q.   When did you come to the hospital?

A.   About 12 years ago.

Q.   Were you here before?

A.   No.

(DR. HAND *checks folder and indicates that she did have a previous hospitalization there.*)

Q.   What brought you to the hospital?

A.   My nerves.

Q.   Do you think you're ready to go home?

A.   Yes, I want to get back home to my family.

Q.   Have you talked to your husband about this?

A.   No, I don't see him much.

Q.   Has he been here to visit?

A.   No.

Q.   Any other reason besides nerves that brought you to the hospital?

A.   No, I don't think so.

Q.   Did you do or say anything?

A.   No.

(PATIENT *was committed for attacking husband. This fact was indicated by* DR. HAND *when the patient was introduced.*)

Q.   If you couldn't go home with your husband, could you go elsewhere?

A.   Maybe someone else in the family, but I got my own home and husband.

(DR. POWELL *indicates he is finished.*)

DR. HAND:

Q.   How do you get along with your husband?

A.   O.K.

Q.   Did you ever hit him?

A.   I don't know; I don't think so.

Q.   Do you recall what you did in the past?

A.   Some things I do.

Q.   How do you get along with people?

A.   O.K.

Q.   Why did you come here?

A.   It was my nerves; they got away from me.

Q.   How did they get away from you?

A.   Oh, I don't know. I had a nervous breakdown.

Q.   How is the world treating you?

A.   O.K.

Q.   Is everybody your friend?

A.   I get along all right.

Q.   Anybody control your mind?

A.   No.

Q.   Can you read others' minds?

A.   No.

Q.   Do people talk behind your back?

A.   No.

Q.   You hear voices?

A.   No.

Q.   Do you talk to the Lord?

A.   No.

Q.   Do you have any future plans?

A.   What do you mean?

Q.   What can we do for you?

A.   Let me go home to my husband.

Q.   Have you talked to him about going home?

A.   No.

Q.   How do you know he wants you?

A.   I know he does. He's my husband.

Q.   When did you hear from him last?

A.   I don't know. He doesn't write.

DR. POWELL   Do you write him?

PATIENT   No.

DR. HAND   Do you think it's normal not to write and see your husband?

PATIENT   [No response.]

DR. HAND   Do you need to be here?

PATIENT   I don't think so.

DR. HAND   Any questions, Dr. Miller?

DR. MILLER   No.

DR. HAND   Dr. Stone?

DR. STONE   No.

DR. HAND   O.K. You can go now, Mrs. _____.

(PATIENT *leaves.*)

DR. HAND   To me, she's a chronic case. She shows no insight. Of course, she was all right here, no acting out.

DR. POWELL   What can we do if her husband doesn't want her?

DR. HAND   Family care placement.

DR. POWELL   There's no hope of her ever being rehabilitated as I can see. I'd like to move her off the ward. She's only taking up a bed and not getting anything. Maybe a county home; she'd be paranoid, probably curse the superintendent, but she's under control.

DR. HAND   We can recommend that she's as stabilized as ever, and is ready for placement, in general, of any kind. That way if they can't get her back to her family, they can try somewhere else. Everybody agree?

(*There is general agreement expressed through nods and "yeas."*)

We have presented these three cases concerning leave requests to illustrate the general manner in which disposition staff handles such requests. To the nonpsychiatric observer in the situation, *explicit* standards or criteria for the decision process were almost nonexistent. The elements the three cases did seem to have in common appeared to be unrelated to questions concerning the patient's present mental condition, the patient's ward behavior, or the expected success regarding the patient's post-hospital performance. In fact, one of the striking aspects of the three cases is the relative ease with which the leaves were granted despite the staff's pessimism concerning post-hospital performance. How can we explain this apparent willingness to release a patient who is not considered well enough to remain out of the hospital?

The main reason for this phenomenon seems to lie in the staff's definition of the seriousness of the staff decision in the situation. That is, the decision to grant a leave is not felt to be so serious as to give the staff members considerable cause for concern. It would seem that the granting of a leave, in light of the pessimistic post-hospital prognosis, would be considered very serious because each error in judgment would put staffing decisions in a questionable light. Would not these errors also raise questions concerning the legitimacy of staff's "quality control" function? Curiously enough, instead of the legitimacy of staff decisions being questioned, their decisions are defined as quite correct, appropriate, and unaffected by errors—i.e., patients who do not "make it" on leave. This seems to take place for several reasons. For one thing, the decision to grant a leave does not indicate the success of the hospital in "producing a finished product." They are not indicating that the patient is well, recovered, or ready to resume her life in the larger society. Thus, they are not evaluating the effectiveness of the hospital's treatment function by putting the stamp of "approval" on the patient's psychological condition. Second, the leave is granted with the understanding that responsible persons will be substituting for the hospital in providing supervision and continuing the patient on her prescribed medication. This feature of the leave also shifts the locus of "blame" for patients who may have some kind of extreme reaction while on leave. That is, though the patient may have been "intact" on leaving the hospital, the particular conditions in the home environment are viewed as the cause of the patient's failure to stay on leave. The demanding mother, the protective father, or the drinking husband can each shoulder the blame for a patient's failure on leave. A third, and by no means unimportant aspect of the leave is that the request is coming from outside the system. Thus, in a sense, no particular staff member is "laying himself on the line" by pushing for a patient's leave. In addition, an interested relative, of whom there are few in number in relation to a large state hospital, can become either a happy relative, by having the leave granted, or an unhappy source of pressure, by taking her request to the superintendent.

Turning to the *discharge* request, we find that the seriousness of the staff decision is much more pronounced. A staff decision granting a discharge does put an official stamp on both the patient's condition and the effectiveness of the hospital treatment program. In a real sense, the staff decision to discharge is a guarantee to the public that a particular patient is ready to "fit in" again. As one physician stated, "It's no joke to discharge a patient. If they're not ready and we turn them loose, we're really responsible for anything they may do." In addition, any judgment by staff on a discharge request inevitably provokes disagreement among staff members. Not only among staff physicians themselves, but among every level of staff having knowledge of the patient in question, there will be divergences of opinion concerning the patient's readiness for discharge. Therefore, no matter whether a discharge request is granted or denied, there will be a residue of disagreement among various staff persons. Thus errors in judgment in this context—i.e., patients who "blow up" after discharge—can come back to haunt the physician who supported the discharge. Staff members who did not support a discharge request for a patient who nevertheless received the discharge and subsequently returned as an "error" will often remind the supporting staff member of his mistaken judgment. This usually comes up in the context of a patient who is seeking a discharge, where one staff member will say: "This case is very similar to Mary Jones' case. You remember how convinced you were that she was ready, and I didn't think so. She got her discharge, and she was back here in three months. This girl will do the same thing if we let her go."

What we find, then, is a rather pronounced conservatism among staff physicians regarding the granting of a discharge request, as compared to a leave request.[7] That is, it is easier to get a leave than a discharge. As a result, it appears that despite the fact that a patient does not closely approach some ideal condition of "wellness," thereby giving the patient a poor post-hospital performance prognosis, he or she is more likely to *leave* the hospital than a patient who more closely approaches some ideal condition of "wellness," but who is requesting a discharge. This appears to be the case because the latter patient is faced with a set of standards that have been redefined to fit the perceived seriousness of the situation.

THE NEED FOR STRUCTURE IN STAFF DECISIONS

Staff definitions regarding leave requests and discharge requests can be viewed as providing a set of implicit standards for making decisions. These standards, however, appear to be somewhat extraneous to the question that is presumably at the heart of the function of staff—namely, "Is this patient well enough to leave the hospital?" But, as we have already suggested, the knowledge necessary to answer this question is not readily available for us in a

---

[7] It is difficult to determine how much of this conservatism is due to the medical theories of mental illness that physicians adhere to and how much is due to the powerlessness of physicians to set the standards for the entire release process.

highly rational, calculable, and predictable manner. How, then, do staff physicians govern their own decisions? Obviously, they must operate within some framework of standards which provides *structure* for the decision-making process. It is this structure that provides the stamp of legitimacy to the staff decision. Again, staff decisions cannot be made without standards or criteria, nor can the standards be "pulled out of a hat," so to speak. The standards must have some credibility, be it relevant knowledge, or "masking" beliefs.

The different staff definitions of seriousness regarding leave and discharge requests are examples of the manner in which *structure* is provided for the decision process. Additional sources from which structure emerges can be found in (1) the potential complexity of the decision—i.e., how much additional work or problems the decision will generate and (2) the strength of the resistance to, or support for, the request by an individual or group in the hospital. Each of these sources of structure are also extraneous to the essential and basic question: "Is this patient well enough to leave the hospital?" Below are examples of the intrusion of these extraneous considerations into the decision process. The text of the entire staff discussion is *not* reported as in the earlier cases in this paper; what we report here is the discussion that crystallized the final decision (all reported discussion took place after each patient was questioned and left the staffing room).

CASE 411

DR. HAND   Well, what shall we do? Dr. Hill and Social Service want her discharged.

DR. CRAIG   I'm not sure about a discharge. Why don't we just give her six months' L.A.?

DR. HAND   If we give her an L.A., she won't get the additional social security money she's got coming. If she doesn't get the money, she can't very well take care of herself.

DR. CRAIG   Well, maybe we ought to discharge her and keep our fingers crossed.

DR. HAND   The main problem is that she gets more money after her discharge. If she runs off to California again we'll just have to go get her. What do you think, Dr. Craig?

DR. CRAIG   They [Social Service] have it all set up.

DR. STONE They expect it, so while they're in the mood, let's do it. I'll go along with them any day.

DR. HAND If there are no objections, then, we'll discharge.

CASE 1141

DR. HAND She's been a good patient here, but I'd be more inclined to give her six months' L.A. instead of a discharge. What do you think, Dr. Powell?

DR. POWELL I'd just discharge her and let her go to Detroit.

DR. HAND Why not just give her an L.A. and let her go to her daughter in Detroit?

DR. POWELL An L.A. out of state!

DR. HAND Oh, yes. There's a lot of red tape going out of state. It would be a lot easier for us to give a discharge. [*Brief pause*]. O.K. We'll discharge her. Any objection?

CASE 75

DR. CRAIG He's not psychotic. He doesn't belong here. A nursing home would be fine, but I think he should be home and his wife should take care of him.

DR. HAND What do you want to do? He's your patient.

DR. CRAIG I want to send him home. Discharge him!

DR. HAND What do you think, Dr. Stone?

DR. STONE He's just a confused old man. He's strong-minded and gives you a hard time on the ward.

DR. HAND His wife doesn't want him. How are we going to discharge him?

DR. CRAIG She's got to take him. It's her responsibility.

DR. HAND I think it's going to be tough. Not that I don't agree with you [DR. CRAIG], but he's been here a long time. It's tough. What do you think, Dr. Powell?

DR. POWELL [*No response*].

DR. CRAIG She's just getting rid of him for forty dollars a month. Let's get him home on L.A. for six months.

CASE 271

DR. HAND Well, what shall we do? He's up for discharge. His brother wants him to go to [*name of state*], but he'd rather stay in [*name of another state*]. What do you think, Dr. Stone?

DR. STONE I think he can go; let's discharge him.

DR. HAND   How can we discharge if he doesn't want to go to his brother? If he'd go to [*out of state*], it's no problem. It's out of state and no work for us. But he wants to go to [*in state*]. That means we have to get a sponsor and give him an L.A.

DR. STONE   Let's forget the discharge then. Give him an L.A. for six months.

DR. HAND   O.K. L.A. for six months. Everyone agree?

These, then, are examples of factors external to the situation which provided the necessary structure that led to a crystallization of the staff decision. In each case, the decision was shaped in terms of its conformability to external conditions, and not to the behavior or mental condition of the patient. This does not mean that the behavior or mental condition of a patient does not enter the staff decision as a major criterion. Clearly, in many of the staffing decisions, psychiatric knowledge applied to the patient's perform- ance at staff becomes the dominant criterion. In fact, the major premise underlying the function of staff is that the "unwell" pa- tient will reveal herself or be revealed. Thus, the "unwell" will not be discharged, while the "well" patient will be discharged. How- ever, we would like to suggest an alternative hypothesis; namely, that under certain limited conditions, the relatively "unwell" patient (as measured by performance at staff) will be more likely to get a discharge than the relatively "well" patient. The suggested explanation for this organization paradox follows.

DISCHARGE: AN ORGANIZATIONAL PARADOX

"Going to staff" is recognized by most patients and staff as a situa- tion that produces a great deal of anxiety for the patients. Pa- tients are expected to perform in a manner that will ensure a favorable decision by the staff. Often the sheer anticipation of going to staff is enough to raise a patient's anxiety so as to make her incapable of giving an adequate performance. What is often overlooked, however, is the fact that going to staff also produces a great deal of anxiety for the attending physician at staff. In ex- ercising their "quality control" function, the physicians are ex- pected to make decisions of considerable importance to patients, the hospital, and the community. However, it is not the decision situation itself that produces the anxiety for staff, but the fact that the decision must be made according to criteria that provide legitimacy for the physician's behavior at staff. The staff physician must provide himself and, by extension, others, with information that attests to the correctness of his decision.

In this situation, the physician is provided with two sources from which he may legitimize his decision. First is the *external* structure, of which we have spoken. Here we find the decision being made in terms of such factors as the amount of staff support there is for a certain decision, the legal complications of the decision, the extent of the family pressure for a decision, and the like. In the absence of any external structure to legitimize the decision, the staff physician is essentially thrown back on his own resources. That is, he must, with the tools of his trade such as knowledge of the dynamics of pathology, make the decision to grant or deny a discharge. Thus, the staff physicians depend upon their available fund of questions which are designed to elicit that information from the patient necessary to make the correct decision. The curious aspect of this second source of legitimization is that basically the staff, through their questioning, depend upon the patients to tell them whether or not they are well enough to receive a discharge. The staff physicians are expected to base their decisions upon an analysis of the patient's responses. All the physician has to work with, then, are his own questions, and the responses of the patient.

In this setting—where there is a relative absence of external legitimation and the physician must depend upon his own resources—we would apply our hypotheses that the relatively "unwell" patient is more likely to get a discharge than the relatively "well" patient. The rationale here is that the "unwell" patient provides *structure* for the situation with her responses, while the "well" patient only increases the already present anxieties of the staff by requiring them to be able to apply additional knowledge to the situation which they do not possess. The situation for these cases would be something like the following.

At staff, the relatively "unwell" patient is confronted with the standard questions of the physicians. During the questioning, the "unwell" patient will provide what we might call a little "pathological content" in some of her answers. That is, she will give some inappropriate answers to questions of orientation, or provide answers that may be psychiatrically interpreted as recognizable symptoms of a certain diagnosed condition. It is significant that this "pathological content" comes to light very early in the questioning process, for the staff's fund of available questions is never really exhausted.

Once the "pathological content" is given by the patient, the staff members are provided with a "foothold" which allows them to exercise their own psychiatric knowledge. Extended discussions take place concerning whether a "manic in remission is really in remission, or only in a modified depressive phase," or "what is the basic difference between some ideal state of mental health and simply manageable symptoms." Thus, the "pathological content" injected by the patient allows the staff to actually *fulfill their "quality control" function in a legitimized manner*. The anxiety that is built into the staffing situation is relieved by the fact that the physicians are actually activating their psychiatric roles and utilizing their specialized knowledge in the decision-making process. In this process of fulfilling their own psychiatric roles and their "quality control" task, the patient is, in a sense, forgotten. That is, the existence of the patient at staff becomes secondary to the resolution of questions and the exchange of ideas which grew out of the "pathological content" introduced by the patient. As a result, the relatively "unwell" patient has created a situation that will predispose the staff to view her discharge request in a "more favorable" light.[8]

The relatively "well" patient at staff is also confronted with the same set of standard questions used by the physicians. However, in response to these questions the "well" patient does not provide that little "pathological content" that the "unwell" patient

[8] It should be kept in mind that we are not speaking of the markedly disturbed patient who also provides the "pathological content" which integrates the staff by allowing them to fulfill their psychiatric roles. Our "unwell" patient is one who is quite "intact," and who gets on well in the hospital. We are not making an independent judgment as to the "sickness" or "wellness" of the patients in question. For our purposes, the "unwell" definition simply applies to those patients who inject "pathological content" into the staffing situation. It should also be clear, however, that we would extend our discussion here to what takes place at staff for patients of psychiatrically determined degrees of "wellness."

does. That is, she is not helping the staff by providing a structure to the situation. Thus, although it may seem that the patient who breezes through staff questioning, by giving appropriate answers to all questions will get a quick and easy decision granting a discharge, it does not appear to work this way. For one thing, the fund of questions used by staff are not the actual criteria for the final decision, but the means by which responses may be elicited and evaluated. The patient who gives appropriate answers to all the questions, then, is depriving the staff of the opportuntiy to exercise their particular staffing function. Because the staff does not receive any structure from the patient, a legitimized final decision cannot be made.

In response to this situation, there is little that staff can do but continue to ask questions in search of structure. As more and more questions are asked, the familiar questions are soon exhausted; to be followed by a "groping" for questions which range from the repetitious to the irrelevant. In addition, as each subsequent question is asked and answered appropriately, the already existing level of anxiety is rapidly magnified. What will generally happen in this situation then, is that as additional questions are asked, the likelihood that the patient will give an inappropriate answer is greatly increased. More important is the fact that when the inappropriate answer is finally forthcoming—an answer that might be overlooked under other conditions—the staff reaction is markedly different from usual staff behavior during the decision-making process. What is indicated by the staff behavior in this situation is a sort of "tension release" effect whereby anxieties of staff members become redirected toward the patient in a highly emotionalized manner.

We will present below a case that illustrates the hypothesis we have suggested. This case involves a discharge request in which the patient provided no structure for the situation, and the nature of staff reaction to the problem.

Case 63

DR. HAND   The next on is _____, a discharge request. She says she can get a lab job in Benton Hospital. Would you tell us something about her, Mrs. Rand [*the patient's ward nurse*]?

MRS. RAND   Well, _____ has been after a discharge for a while now. I asked Dr. Powell if we shouldn't try, and he said maybe we should. I think it's a shame to keep her here. She's a very bright girl, and she's really learned her lab work. Lately, she has refused to take her medicine. She says it doesn't help her; and besides, she says she doesn't need us to take her medicine.

DR. HAND   I have a note here from her work supervisor indicating that she works well in the lab and has picked up a great deal.

DR. MILLER   Shouldn't we wait for Dr. Powell before we handle her case?

DR. HAND   No, he won't be able to make it today, so we'll have to go on without him. Will you show her in, Dr. Craig?

(PATIENT *enters.*)

DR. HAND:

Q.   I see where you want to get a job at Benson Hospital.

A.   Yes, I talked with their lab director last time I was in Benton and he was interested.

Q.   Do you think you would like lab work as a permanent job?

A.   Oh, yes, I enjoy my work here very much.

Q.   It's really not easy work running all those tests. Are you bothered by the blood tests?

A.   No, I don't mind them.

Q.   Do you know who the governor of _____ is?

A.   [*Appropriately answered*].

Q.   Do you remember when you first came to Riverview?

A.   [*Appropriately answered*].

DR. CRAIG:

Q.   How do you know you'll get a job at Benton if you're discharged?

A.   I told you I talked to the lab director, and he was interested.

Q.   Suppose he's not as interested as he appeared to you? Where will you work if you can't get in at Benton Hospital?

A.   I think I know my lab work well enough to get a lab technician job somewhere.

Q.   Well, let's see how much lab work you really know.

(DR. CRAIG *asks the* PATIENT *more questions pertaining to various procedures and lab tests. After the last response,* DR. CRAIG *indicates that the* PATIENT *does know her lab work.*)

DR. HAND:

Q.   How do you get along with the other patients?

A.   Not very well. I have a few close friends, but I don't socialize with the other patients.

Q.   What bothers you about the other patients?

A. Oh, I don't know. I just don't like living in the hospital.

Q. Do you think we've helped you while you've been here?

A. No, I don't.

Q. What kind of treatment have you had here?

A. Lobotomy and shock.

Q. Do you think it's helped you or tortured you?

A. I think it's tortured me.

(This response brings a stir from others present at staff.)

Q. You mean that we did these things just to torture you?

A. Oh, no, I'm sure that when they give shock they mean to help. I don't think they have.

DR. STONE:

Q. Besides not liking it here, why do you want to go to work?

A. For one thing, I want to start earning my own money, and making my own way.

Q. If you want to make money, we can probably find plenty of opportunities for you to make money right here.

A. You mean like washing cars. I'm already doing that.

Q. *[in an annoyed tone]* No, I don't mean washing cars. You could probably work full-time in the lab right here on a work placement.

A. I already asked Dr. Galt about an opening in histology, and he said there wasn't any. Anyway, I'd do much better if the hospital would free me.

DR. HAND:

Q. What do you mean, "free you"?

A. Well, it would be just like the other work placements I've had. You're never really free.

(It was at this point in the staffing session that the observer noted the beginnings of the change in staff behavior. The patient's response about "never really being free," was followed by the exchange of glances among the physicians. These glances indicated that they had, so to speak, "picked up the scent." Staff participation at this point no longer followed the orderly procedure of the staff director asking individual members if they had any questions. The physicians spoke whenever they wished, sometimes cutting in on each other, and sometimes several speaking at the same time. The normal speaking tone vanished as pronouncements and accusations were directed at the patient.)

Q. But if you stayed here on a work placement you'd be free to come and go on your own time. It would be just like a job.

A. No. You would still be controlling me if I stayed here.

DR. CRAIG: [cutting in]

Q. Do you mean we control your mind here?

A. You may not control my mind, but I really don't have a mind of my own.

Q. How about if we gave you a work placement in _____; would you be free then? That's far away from here.

A. Any place I went it would be the same set-up as it is here. You're never really free; you're still a patient, and everyone you work with knows it. It's tough to get away from the hospital's control.

DR. STONE [cutting in] That's the most paranoid statement I ever heard.

MRS. RAND How can you say that, [patient's first name]? That doesn't make any sense. [nurse is standing at this point] It's just plain crazy to say we can control your mind.

(NURSE RAND turns to DR. STONE who is looking at her.)

MRS. RAND [still standing] I had no idea she was that sick. She sure had me fooled. [turning to PATIENT again] You're just not well enough for a discharge, [first name], and you had better realize that.

DR. STONE She's obviously paranoid.

(Immediately following Dr. Stone's remark, Dr. Craig stood up, followed by social worker Holmes. Dr. Stone himself then stood up to join the others, including Nurse Rand, who had been standing for some time. It should be noted that this took place without any indication from Dr. Hand, the staff director, that the interview was completed. He then turned to the patient and dismissed her. After the patient left, the standing staff members engaged themselves in highly animated discussion. Nurse Rand was involved in making general apologies for having indicated support of the patient's discharge request at the beginning of the staff meeting. Drs. Stone and Craig were engaged in monologues interpreting and reinterpreting the patient's statements. Amid the confusion, Dr. Hand managed to comment, "I guess there's no need to vote on her; it's quite clear.")[9]

[9] Although it may appear that the picture of confusion presented here is quite overdrawn, the observer could not help but respond to the very marked aspects of this staff meeting as compared to any other staff meeting he attended. If the descriptive account takes on the aspects of a caricature, it is primarily because of the observed departures from the expected.

After leaving staff, the observer returned to the ward to speak with the patient in question. She was very disappointed and bitter. Among her remarks was her accusation that Dr. Powell had never really wanted her to get a discharge, for if he did, he would have been at staff to support her request. However, the patient did appear to show some insight into what had taken place at staff. She made the following remark: "I did learn something from that staff, though. If I ever get a chance to go again, I'll keep my big mouth shut, and I'll lie like hell. This time I said what I really felt, and look what happened."

The decision process described in these case documents indicate the varied criteria that influence staffing decisions. In the cases presented, decision criteria were identified that were related to such matters as the source of and support for the release request, the locus of responsibility for "errors" in staff decisions, and the degree of anxiety generated by staff's inability to find criteria within the staffing situation itself. In each case, the criteria are not centrally relevant to the degree of illness of the patient, but are related to a number of social conditions which indicate that psychiatric decisions are made within a social system context.

These findings show important similarities to those reported in studies on the prehospital career of the patient. In the commitment process, the family member was a central figure whose request for commitment greatly increased the likelihood of commitment. Linn[10] reported that the spouse and parents were more likely to commit than any other relative or non-family agent. Goffman[11] also pointed to the part played by the family member in moving the person from a civil to patient status, which he has called the betrayal cycle. The greater the involvement of the family member in the commitment process, the easier the task of hospital psychiatric agents, in that there will be greater legitimation of the commitment decision. This same pattern is clearly at work in our data on the release process. Under conditions where a family member is eager to have a patient released and is pressing for such a release, staff decisions are likely to meet the family requests. This

[10] Erwin L. Linn, "Agents, Timing, and Events Leading to Mental Hospitalization," *Human Organization,* 20 (Summer 1961), 92–98.

[11] Erving Goffman, *Asylums* (New York: Doubleday-Anchor, 1961), 137–141.

occurs precisely because the family shoulders the responsibility for the patient and thereby relieves the hospital of responsibility.

Hospital staff who lack the power to control the release process are nonetheless forced to establish criteria for making decisions concerning the release of patients. The criteria established are more likely to be adaptations to the internal and external pressures facing the staff, rather than serious efforts to assess the mental status of the patient being considered for release.

The medical staff's search for a stable and legitimate basis for making decisions about release is not very different from the search behavior of patients trying to discover how to get out of the hospital (as described in the previous chapter). Both physicians and patients feel that they are not in control of the situation that confronts them. They share a vulnerability to those "forces" which they do not fully understand, but which are responsible for patients being in the hospital and for physicians being thrust into the role of caretakers.

What hospital staff and patients do to each other and to themselves in the process of believing that there is a disease called a mental illness constitutes the special madness that they share.

8

Victims and Caretakers: A Final Note on Madness in American Society

The main objective of this book has been to describe and understand the social structure of a mental hospital. We have maintained the view that the internal life of a mental hospital results from the special relationship that exists between the hospital and the larger society. This relationship finds expression in the reasons why people are put in mental hospitals in the first place and in the limited power of the hospital to do much beyond making sure that patients stay there. A mental hospital is a place to put people who have been rejected by their families and communities. This fact is "hidden" from society and from patients' families by a variety of theories that define mental illness as a disease that resides in the body of the afflicted person.

To suggest that mental patients are victims is not to say that they are without personal problems. They do experience severe *problems of living* that involve interpersonal difficulties with family, friends, and employers. Many also experience life under conditions of extensive deprivation, both economic and emotional. Deprived of sufficient economic resources, most mental patients have spent a large part of their pre-patient lives, as children and adults, trying to cope with this deprivation. They begin life, therefore, as victims of a system of inequality of resources and life chances that places them at the bottom of society with little prospect for improvement. When confronted with problems of living, they are without the resources that can help them to cope. Their own families and friends often suffer similar deprivations, and hence, cannot help in getting others over especially difficult periods.

Commitment to a mental hospital has less to do with having a disease called "mental illness" than with being without sufficient resources to deal with problems that are experienced by many people, most of whom do not become mental patients. Mental illness is therefore best understood as a social process rather than as a medical one. It is a process that starts with unusual or problematic behaviors and ends with everyone, including the victim, believing that someone has a mental illness and requires hospitalization. Let us now consider that process.

Mental Illness as Social Deviance

The early involvement of sociologists in the study of mental illness was concerned mainly with finding those characteristics of the social environment that were associated with functional disorders. Special attention was given to those social conditions which provided a good fit with psychological theories of mental illness, with the result that sick personalities were found to abound in areas of social disorganization. Thus, high rates of illness were found in the central areas of the city characterized by rooming-house dwellings, transients, and fleeting social relationships.[1] The mentally ill as compared to the "normal" were often found to be social isolates, less involved in the mainstream of social life.[2]

Much of the early work was built upon an idealized view of the sacred, pre-urban society with stable social relationships that bind men together, and to a cultural tradition of shared beliefs. The contrasting image of the urban society is one of anonymity, alienation from self and others, and self-interest as a main principle of social life.[3] These assumptions about life in the pre-industrial society and mental illness were challenged by the work of Goldhammer and

[1] Robert E. F. Faris and H. Warren Dunham, *Mental Disorders in Urban Areas* (Chicago: University of Chicago Press, 1939).

[2] E. Gartley Jaco, "The Social Isolation Hypothesis and Schizophrenia," *American Sociological Review,* 19 (October 1954), 567–77; and Melvin Kohn and John Clausen, "Social Isolation and Schizophrenia," *American Sociological Review,* 20 (June 1955), 265–73.

[3] Edward Shils, "Daydreams and Nightmares: Reflections on the Criticism of Mass Culture," *Sewanee Review,* Vol. 65 (Autumn 1957).

Marshall [4] and Eaton and Weil.[5] The former study was an examination of admission rates for state hospitals in Massachusetts, comparing rates from 1840 to 1860, and for the United States as a whole in 1940. Goldhammer and Marshall's analysis revealed no significant increase in psychosis over time, thereby failing to give general support for the hypothesis that the greater complexity of modern living gives rise to higher rates of mental illness. The Eaton and Weil study also represents, in a sense, an analysis of the relation between social and cultural complexity and mental illness. It presents a picture of the Hutterite community as one of a consistent, well-integrated culture, having few internal contradictions and characterized by homogeneity of values. There is virtually no differentiation of class, income, or standard of living, for the Hutterites are organized on a communal basis. In this setting, in which the relative absence of mental disorders might be expected, the authors do not find the subjects to be immune from mental disorders, although their rates are considerably lower than those for the U.S. population as a whole.

Sociologists turned their attention from the search for etiological factors in the development of functional mental disorders to an examination of the social institution of insanity.[6] They detached themselves, so to speak, from actual participation in the cultural pattern itself, standing outside the process and observing its operation. Rather than seeking to develop sociological theories which provide supportive evidence for psychological theories of schizophrenia and psychoneurosis, sociologists become more concerned with the manner in which such illness designations were assigned to persons and how such designations influenced the future course of illness. Major concern now shifted to how the mentally ill were identified as ill, how they did or did not find their way to becoming patients, how life in the closed communities of patients affected their disorder, how patients move from a state of illness to wellness, and how, having returned to the larger community, ex-patients are able to shed the stigma of their former life.

[4] Herbert Goldhammer and Herbert Marshall, *Psychosis and Civilization* (New York: The Free Press, 1953).

[5] Joseph W. Eaton and Robert J. Weil, *Culture and Mental Disorders* (New York: The Free Press, 1955).

[6] Elaine Cumming and John Cumming, *Closed Ranks* (Cambridge, Mass.: Harvard University Press, 1957).

In 1951, Lemert presented an approach to understanding mental disorders which emphasized the importance of interpersonal relationships in the family and community in defining deviant behavior as mental illness. As Lemert put it:

> It would probably be the consensus of most trained observers of mental disorders that psychotic deviation as described in formal psychiatric categories is not in itself the reason for collective action to bring mentally disturbed persons under restraint. Rather, it is the highly visible deviations of the psychotic person from the norms of his group, placing strain upon other persons, which excite his family or the community and cause them to take formal, legal action against him.[7]

Thus, collective action by the family or community to commit a disturbed person will be the product of the stressful nature of the deviance and the tolerance of the group for such deviance. A similar view was expressed by Clausen and Yarrow[8] in a paper dealing with the ways in which patients find their way to the mental hospital. They sought to identify those persons and agencies that play decisive roles in defining a patient's difficulties and who aid (or hinder) effective action in getting persons to the hospital.

The relevance of a deviancy perspective for understanding how persons become identified as mentally ill is emphasized by recent surveys that have attempted to measure the prevalence rates of mental illness in the general population. These surveys have obtained very high estimates of the extent of emotional impairment among nonhospitalized persons.[9] Such findings raise the question of precisely what factors distinguish an emotionally impaired hospitalized person from an emotionally impaired nonhospitalized person. The answer to this question can perhaps be best pursued by looking at the social processes involved in the identification and classification of a person into the *socially defined role* of "mentally ill."

The pre-hospital career of the mental patient can be divided into three discernible stages. The stages are interdependent to the extent

---

[7] Edwin M. Lemert, *Social Pathology* (New York: McGraw-Hill, 1951).

[8] John A. Clausen and Marion R. Yarrow, "Paths to the Mental Hospital," *The Journal of Social Issues,* 11 (December 1955), 25–33.

[9] Leo Srole et al., *Mental Health in the Metropolis: The Midtown Manhattan Study* (New York: McGraw-Hill, 1962).

of the order of their occurrence, but not with respect to the absolute necessity that all three stages take place in the pre-hospital career.[10] Let us examine each stage in terms of how it might increase the probability of becoming identified as mentally ill.

THE REACTIONS TO "UNUSUAL" BEHAVIOR WHICH RESULT IN A DEFINITION OF DEVIANCY

Persons find themselves in deviant social roles when other persons respond to their "peculiar" or "unusual" behavior as inappropriate to a situation or not in keeping with a shared standard of conduct, or failure to meet the expectations of some social role. It is the response of the group, therefore, that places someone in a deviant role. It should also be clear, however, that such a view of deviancy also makes it possible for the originally "peculiar" behavior of persons to be transformed into familiar, expected, and accepted behavior, thereby avoiding definitions of deviancy. Cumming and Cumming,[11] in their study of community reaction to mental illness, describe the response to deviance in terms of denial, isolation, and insulation. Interviews with wives of mental patients reveal a process of continuous "groping" for definitions of the behavior of their husbands which will help them to interpret and explain the behavior.[12] A similar analysis using hospital documents rather than interviewing family members indicated that families tend to react to a totality of "unusual" behaviors rather than a specific type of behavior, and that the family's tolerance for deviance decreases with close familial relationships.[13] Such indications of the great ambiguity in defining "unusual" behavior points to the importance that having a vocabulary of explanations may have for defining deviance. Such vocabularies may be part of the idea systems of a family or they may be provided by other persons or agencies in the community.

[10] Other stages and sequences of events are, of course, also possible. We are here attempting to present one possible sequence.

[11] Cumming and Cumming, *Closed Ranks,* pp. 587–608.

[12] Charlotte G. Schwartz, "Perspectives on Deviance—Wives' Definitions of Their Husbands' Mental Illness," *Psychiatry,* 20 (August 1957), 257–91.

[13] Erwin L. Linn, "Agents, Timing, and Events Leading to Mental Hospitalization," *Human Organization,* 20 (Summer 1961), 92–98.

THE CONSTRAINTS UPON THE DEVIANT TO TAKE ON A DEVIANT ROLE

The existence of a vocabulary for defining certain types of behavior can be seen as a factor that influences a person to take on a deviant role. The deviant individuals themselves may possess such vocabularies which they use to define their behavior, or they may be found among persons of certain educational and occupational characteristics, or they may be found in the existence of mental health agencies and facilities in the community. A recent study reported how differential use of a psychiatric out-patient clinic serving children is related *not* to the incidence or prevalence of mental illness in the child population, but to the extent to which the mental health innovation had been communicated throughout the community and had received a favorable reaction.[14]

An additional element constraining deviants to take on a deviant role is what Scheff [15] has called the special vulnerability of deviants to the suggestions and influence of others. He has offered the hypothesis that because the "primary deviant may be profoundly confused, anxious, and ashamed," he will be suggestible to the cues and reactions of others to him. These cues may be part of the traditional stereotype of insanity that may also be a part of the deviant's vocabulary for explaining his own behavior. Scheff suggests that "once a person has been placed in a deviant status there are rewards for conforming to the deviant role, and punishment for not conforming to the deviant role.[16]

THE MANNER IN WHICH THE DEVIANT ROLE ITSELF SHAPES THE SUBSEQUENT BEHAVIORS OF THE DEVIANT

Once the deviant role is occupied, the deviant is often cut off from "normal" role relationships, from "normal" responses to social

[14] Edna E. Raphael, "Community Structure and Acceptance of Psychiatric Aid," *American Journal of Sociology*, 69 (January 1964), 340–59.

[15] Thomas J. Scheff, "The Role of the Mentally Ill and the Dynamics of Mental Disorder: A Research Framework," *Sociometry*, 26 (December 1963), 436–53.

[16] Ibid.

situations, and from the supportive relationships of the group in time of stress. In a study of deviance in four cultural groups, Mizruchi and Perrucci[17] suggested that deviants in cultural groups that are organized around normative systems which are characterized as proscriptive, inflexible, and unintegrated are more likely to exhibit extreme reactions to deviance (i.e., problem drinking and alcoholism) than members of cultural groups that are organized around prescriptive, flexible, and integrative normative systems. This bears a striking resemblance to our earlier discussion of families with a low tolerance for deviance, and suggests that deviants may not be able to shed a deviant role because they are outside the group and because the group's normative system does not tolerate "gray" areas of behavior. The findings of Glass[18] on combat neurosis (as reported in Scheff) suggest a similar pattern on the function of the group context in allowing for deviants to shift from deviant to nondeviant roles. Combat neuroses among soldiers are often self-terminating if the soldier is kept with the unit, but those who are removed from their unit to a hospital often go on to become more seriously impaired.

Thus, the pre-hospital career of the mental patient is shaped by the social context in which deviance occurs, is identified, and in which the response to it takes place. The deviant role itself continues to influence the response of others to the deviant throughout the remainder of his deviant career. Psychiatric decisions concerning commitment, which are often made under conditions of uncertainty, are more likely to err on the side of judging a well person sick than a sick person well.[19] Operating with such conservative decision rules ("When in doubt, commit") will undoubtedly generate some anxiety among decision makers and for the institutions of decision making. Under such conditions of anxiety and doubt, attempts at justification or rationalization of the decisions are undertaken. Such justifi-

[17] Ephraim H. Mizruchi and Robert Perrucci, "Norm Qualities and Differential Effects of Deviant Behavior: An Exploratory Analysis," *American Sociological Quarterly,* 27 (June 1962), 391–99.

[18] Albert J. Glass (as reported in Scheff), "Psychotherapy in the Combat Zone," in *Symposium on Stress* (Army Medical Service Graduate School, 1953).

[19] Thomas J. Scheff, "Decision Rules, Types of Error, and Their Consequences in Medical Diagnosis," in Fred Massarik and Philburn Ratoosh, *Mathematical Explorations in Behavioral Science* (Homewood, Ill.: 1965).

cation processes can be seen at work in Goffman's description of how the support of closest kin is sought in order to legitimize the commitment decision.[20] In addition to the search for support for the decision process, once a patient is committed, there are elaborate organizational norms and rules which serve to discredit the patient and raise questions concerning the credibility of anything he may say. The patient folder often becomes an extensive dossier of events testifying to the illness of the patient rather than balanced reports representing a sampling of behavior. In Riverview Hospital, "behavior notes" on the patient were recorded only about fights, sleepless nights, inappropriate content in speech, and the like. With the passage of time, idle observations, hypotheses and allegations injected into a patient's folder become transformed into "factual" material when read by physicians who are trying to make decisions concerning patients.

After commitment, the course and treatment of a patient's "illness" becomes so intertwined with the social and cultural patterns in the hospital itself that it becomes impossible to differentiate adaptive role behavior from the particular problems that were presumed to be the cause of the commitment.

As stated in Chapter Two, then, it is easier to understand what occurs in mental hospitals if one assumes that the people who are there are victims of a social process which creates deviance rather than medical problems. This assumption also facilitates one's understanding of the special function of caretaking institutions such as mental hospitals and the special problems faced by caretakers therein.

Caretakers and Caretaking Institutions

Becoming defined as someone whose problems with living are intolerable to a family or community is an experience not limited to mental patients. The aged, vagrants, drunks, and problem children all share with mental patients a judgment that they create too much trouble to continue as members of society. They interfere with otherwise smooth-functioning and orderly families or communities and must, therefore, be removed and placed in other set-

[20] Erving Goffman, *Asylums* (New York: Doubleday-Anchor, 1961).

tings. People who have increasing difficulty in finding a place in a society that tries to run like an efficient production system find themselves in some sort of caretaking institution such as a mental hospital, nursing home, orphanage, or detention center.

The creation of caretaking institutions permits the *total exclusion* from the larger society of persons with problems of living. The problems are apparently believed to require total exclusion rather than assistance, care, treatment, counseling, etc. while their bearers remain *in* society. Closely connected with the process of total exclusion is the *objectification* of a class of persons who are presumed to share some common problem or disability. Objectification renders this class of persons as objects for study and leads to a decrease in the perception of their humanness. It deprives them of ordinary human and civil rights because they are a class of persons to whom and for whom things are done in order to assist them with their problem.

The fullest form of objectification is achieved when the class of persons with problems is provided with a class of professionals whose expertise and calling makes them the caretakers of the problem people. Thus, we have social workers for the poor, psychiatrists for the mentally ill, psychologists for youthful offenders, and gerontologists for the aged. These professionals are expected to use their expert knowledge on behalf of the problem group they serve, and as such, they develop a vested interest in the continued social definition of some members of society as exhibiting a particular affliction. They are, therefore, interested in helping people while they are in the problem category, in helping them to move on to a nonproblem category, and in replenishing the category with new members who must be "found" in the larger society.

One of the main tasks of caretaker-professionals is to develop a body of scientifically based "theory" which purports to explain why a person becomes a particular type of problem, and tells what to do with him while he is a problem and how to help him stop being a problem. Despite their objective-scientific aspect, these "theories" make a moral judgment on the problem and establish who is responsible for its creation and cure. In the case of the mentally ill, there has developed a theory of *victim responsibility* in the sense that elements connected with a person's psycho-social history are responsible for the illness in the first place. Cure, moreover, also requires victim responsibility in the sense of an awareness of one's psycho-social history and a willingness to change some aspect of one's behavior and self-concept. This view of victim responsibility is a feature of the medical model of mental illness which dominates our mental hospitals.

Thus, the emergence of caretaking institutions requires four elements: (1) the total exclusion of the victims from normal society; (2) the objectification of the victims, which denies their humanness and renders them powerless to resist their own "care and treatment"; (3) caretaker-professionals who are in charge of the victims; and (4) a theory of victim responsibility for either their condition or their cure. With the emergence of caretaking institutions comes potential conflict between the segments of society that benefit from a total exclusion of people with problems of living, and the caretaker-professionals who provide the justification necessary for their exclusion. Conflict is avoided or resolved by a division of spheres of control. Caretaker-professionals have autonomy over the internal life of the institution, while agents of the larger society control the basic resources of the institution including the patient population—that is, they have power over who is admitted and released.

A final characteristic of caretaking institutions, which was discussed in Chapter Two, is the stigma that caretakers come to share with patients. Although the sources of the phenomenon of shared stigma are unclear, its immediate causes are related to the personal and professional marginality of caretakers. One is tempted to view such marginality as a necessary part of the entire process of victimization. If, as we assumed, members of society need to feel justified before they sanction the process of total exclusion—and they also expect caretaker-professionals to provide them with such justifying beliefs—it is possible that attempts to discredit the caretakers are designed to prevent them from upsetting the balance of power by intruding upon the decision areas concerning admission and discharge. In addition, such attempts seem designed to maintain a strict separation of political decisions from scientific ones. Despite the common belief that people get into and out of hospitals for scientifically based reasons, our view of mental illness suggests that these decisions are political in the sense that persons with limited resources (including limited power) are victimized by their families and agencies of their community. To give caretaker-professionals more influence over admission and release decisions would shift the balance away from the political basis of victimization.

Throughout this book we have viewed mental patients as victims rather than disease-carriers, and have maintained that patients and their caretakers are bound together by a common stigma and common powerlessness that has a unique effect on the internal social structure of the hospital. If most mental patients could get along quite well outside of the hospital, as I believe, how is it possible to reduce the hospital population to that relatively small number of people for whom no alternative seems possible?

In one respect, there already exists a reversal of the trend of expanding patient populations. The community mental health movement has been successful in keeping large numbers of people in their homes and communities while they receive some medical-psychiatric assistance on an out-patient basis. The present strength of this movement is its economic advantage insofar as it has reduced the costs of supporting a growing hospital population. The movement, however, still lacks a strong theoretical basis for reexamining the whole concept of mental illness as a disease that resides in the afflicted person.

What is required is for the community mental health movement to embrace a view whereby the clients are seen as people without resources for living in a demanding society, without knowledge of their legal rights, and without the ability to resist the efforts of the state to stigmatize them (out-patient status is not exactly a reward) and hospitalize them against their will. When this view is accepted, and when its proponents are strong enough to defeat the proponents of the mental-illness-as-disease theory, then it will be possible to begin the search for ways to limit the power of the state against the individual.

Index